ITI International Team for Implantology

T0093827

ITI Treatment Guide
Volume 12

ITI
Treatment
Guide

Editors:
N. Donos, S. Barter, D. Wismeijer

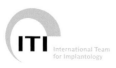

Authors:
M. Roccuzzo
A. Sculean

Volume 12

Peri-Implant Soft-Tissue Integration and Management

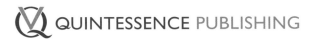 QUINTESSENCE PUBLISHING

Berlin | Chicago | Tokyo
Barcelona | London | Milan | Mexico City | Moscow | Paris | Prague | Seoul | Warsaw
Beijing | Istanbul | Sao Paulo | Zagreb

German National Library CIP Data

The German National Library has listed this publication in the German National Bibliography. Detailed bibliographical data are available at http://dnb.ddb.de.

QUINTESSENCE PUBLISHING

© 2021 Quintessenz Verlags-GmbH
Ifenpfad 2 – 4, 12107 Berlin, Germany
www.quintessence-publishing.com

All rights reserved. This book or any part thereof may not be reproduced, stored in a retrieval system, or transmitted in any form or by any means, whether electronic, mechanical, photocopying, or otherwise, without prior written permission of the publisher.

Illustrations:	Ute Drewes, Basel (CH), www.drewes.ch
Copyediting:	Triacom Dental, Barendorf (DE), www.triacom.com
Graphic concept:	Wirz Corporate AG, Zürich (CH)
Production:	Juliane Richter, Janina Kuhn, Berlin (DE)
Printer:	Grafički zavod Hrvatske Mičevečka ulica 7 HR-10000 Zagreb, Croatia www.gzh.hr

Printed in Croatia
ISBN: 978-1-78698-101-1

The materials offered in the ITI Treatment Guide are for educational purposes only and intended as a step-by-step guide to the treatment of a particular case and patient situation. These recommendations are based on the conclusions of the ITI Consensus Conferences and, as such, are in line with the ITI treatment philosophy. These recommendations, nevertheless, represent the opinions of the authors. Neither the ITI nor the authors, editors, or publishers make any representation or warranty for the completeness or accuracy of the published materials and as a consequence do not accept any liability for damages (including, without limitation, direct, indirect, special, consequential, or incidental damages or loss of profits) caused by the use of the information contained in the ITI Treatment Guide. The information contained in the ITI Treatment Guide cannot replace an individual assessment by a clinician and its use for the treatment of patients is therefore the sole responsibility of the clinician.

The inclusion of or reference to a particular product, method, technique or material relating to such products, methods, or techniques in the ITI Treatment Guide does not represent a recommendation or an endorsement of the values, features, or claims made by its respective manufacturers.

All rights reserved. In particular, the materials published in the ITI Treatment Guide are protected by copyright. Any reproduction, whether in whole or in part, without the publisher's prior written consent is prohibited. The information contained in the published materials can itself be protected by other intellectual property rights. Such information may not be used without the prior written consent of the respective intellectual property right owner.

Some of the manufacturer and product names referred to in this publication may be registered trademarks or proprietary names, even though specific reference to this fact is not made. Therefore, the appearance of a name without designation as proprietary is not to be construed as a representation by the publisher that it is in the public domain.

The tooth identification system used in this ITI Treatment Guide is that of the FDI World Dental Federation.

The ITI Mission is ...

"... to serve the dental profession by providing a growing global network for life-long learning in implant dentistry through comprehensive quality education and innovative research to the benefit of the patient."

Preface

The field of implant dentistry has developed significantly in recent years. As a result, practitioners are faced with higher demand as well as expectations from their patients, not only in terms of successful implant treatment but also the long-term esthetics of the final result. At the same time, the growing number of patients with soft-tissue-related problems is an undeniable reality.

This volume therefore provides readers with guidance and reference material for the treatment of patients with mucogingival deformities. Its aim is to reduce the risk of biological and esthetic complications around dental implants, and to ensure predictable and stable long-term treatment outcomes.

As with every ITI Treatment Guide, this volume illustrates clinical approaches to peri-implant soft-tissue integration and management, step by step, in a variety of clinical situations.

We hope this volume provides clinicians support and orientation towards optimal long-term maintenance of peri-implant soft-tissue health and esthetics.

N. Donos   S. Barter   D. Wismeijer

Acknowledgments

The authors would like to express their gratitude to Dr. Kati Benthaus for her excellent support in the preparation and coordination of this Treatment Guide. We would also like to thank Ms. Ute Drewes for the professional illustrations, Ms. Janina Kuhn (Quintessence Publishing) for the typesetting and for the coordination of the production workflow and Mr. Per N. Döhler (Triacom Dental) for the language editing. We also acknowledge Institut Straumann AG, the corporate partner of the ITI, for its continuing support.

Editors and Authors

Editors:

Nikolaos Donos
    DDS, MS, FHEA, FDSRC, PhD
    Professor, Head and Chair, Periodontology and
    Implant Dentistry
    Head of Clinical Research
    Institute of Dentistry, Barts and The London School
    of Medicine and Dentistry
    Queen Mary University of London
    Turner Street
    London E1 2AD
    United Kingdom
    n.donos@qmul.ac.uk

Stephen Barter
    BDS, MSurgDent, RCS
    Specialist in Oral Surgery
    Honorary Senior Clinical Lecturer/Consultant Oral
    Surgeon
    Centre for Oral Clinical Research
    Institute of Dentistry, Barts and The London School
    of Medicine and Dentistry
    Turner Street
    London E1 2AD
    United Kingdom
    s.barter@qmul.ac.uk

Daniel Wismeijer
    Professor, DMD
    Oral Implantology and Prosthetic Dentistry
    Private Practice
    Zutphensestraatweg 26
    6955 AH Ellecom
    Netherlands
    Danwismeijer@gmail.com

Authors:

Mario Roccuzzo
    DMD, Dr med dent
    Private practice (periodontology)
    Corso Tassoni 14
    10143 Torino (TO)
    Italy
    mroccuzzo@icloud.com

Anton Sculean
    Professor, Dr med dent, Dr h c, MSc
    Executive Director and Chairman
    Department of Periodontology
    University of Bern
    School of Dental Medicine
    Freiburgstrasse 7
    3010 Bern
    Switzerland
    anton.sculean@zmk.unibe.ch

Contributors

Sofia Aroca
Dr med dent, PhD
Private practice
35, Rue Franklin
78100 Saint Germain en Laye
France
sofiaaroca@me.com

Paolo Casentini
DDS, Dr med dent
Private practice
Via Anco Marzio 2
20123 Milano (MI)
Italy
paolocasentini@fastwebnet.it

Raffaele Cavalcanti
DDS, PhD
Adjunct Professor of Periodontology University of
Catania, CLMOPD, Via S. Sofia 78, 95123 Catania
(CT), Italy
and
Private practice
Studio Odontoiatrico Associato Cavalcanti & Venezia
(periodontology, implantology, oral surgery)
Via Giuseppe Posca 15
70124 Bari (BA)
Italy
raffaelecavalcanti@gmail.com

Nikolaos Donos
DDS, MS, FHEA, FDSRC, PhD
Professor, Head and Chair, Periodontology and
Implant Dentistry
Head of Clinical Research
Institute of Dentistry, Barts and The London School
of Medicine and Dentistry
Queen Mary University of London
Turner Street
London E1 2AD
United Kingdom
n.donos@qmul.ac.uk

Daniel Etienne
Dr chir dent, MSc
Private practice
1, Avenue Bugeaud
75116 Paris
France
etienne@paro-implant.com

Jason R Gillespie
BS DDS MS
Private prac:ce (Prosthodon:cs)
105 W El Prado Dr
San Antonio, TX 78212-2024
United States of America
jason@gillespie.dental

Alfonso Gil
DDS, MS, PhD
Resident Physician
Clinic of Reconstructive Dentistry
Center of Dental Medicine
University of Zurich
Plattenstrasse 11
8032 Zurich
Switzerland
alfonso.gil@zzm.uzh.ch

Christoph Hämmerle
Professor, Dr med dent, Dr h c
Chair
Clinic of Reconstructive Dentistry
Center of Dental Medicine
University of Zurich
Plattenstrasse 11
8032 Zurich
Switzerland
christoph.hammerle@zzm.uzh.ch

Vincenzo Iorio-Siciliano
DDS, MS, PhD
Department of Periodontology
University of Naples Federico II
Via Sergio Pansini 5
80131 Napoli (NA)
Italy
enzois@libero.it

Ronald Jung
Professor, Dr med dent, PhD
Head, Oral Implantology
Clinic of Reconstructive Dentistry
Center of Dental Medicine
University of Zurich
Plattenstrasse 11
8032 Zurich
Switzerland
ronald.jung@zzm.uzh.ch

Eduardo Lorenzana
DDS, MSc
Private practice (periodontology)
3519 Paesano's Parkway
Suite 103
San Antonio, TX 78231-1266
United States of America
drlorenzana@yahoo.com

Neil MacBeth
BDS, MFGDP, MGDS RCS, MFDS RCS, FFGDP (UK),
MSc, FDS RCS (Rest Dent), CDLM, RAF
Consultant in Restorative Dentistry –
Defence Primary Health Care
Clinical Senior Lecturer in Periodontology
Institute of Dentistry,
Queen Mary University of London
Institute of Dentistry, Barts and
The London School of Medicine and Dentistry
Turner Street
London E1 2AD
United Kingdom
n.d.macbeth@qmul.ac.uk

Kurt Riewe
DDS
Private practice, Stone Oak Dental
335 E Sonterra Blvd
Suite 150
San Antonio, TX 78258-4295
United States of America
kurt.riewe@gmail.com

Shakeel Shahdad
BDS, MMedSc, FDS RCSEd, FDS (Rest. Dent.)
RCSEd, DDS, FDT FEd
Consultant in Restorative Dentistry
Barts Health NHS Trust
The Royal London Dental Hospital
and
Honorary Clinical Professor in Oral Rehabilitation
and Implantology
Barts and The London School of Medicine
and Dentistry
Queen Mary University of London
Turner Street
London, E1 1DE
United Kingdom
shakeel.shahdad@nhs.net

Daniel Thoma
Professor, Dr med dent
Vice-Chairman
Head, Reconstructive Dentistry
Clinic of Reconstructive Dentistry
Center of Dental Medicine
Vice Chairman, Center for Dental Medicine
University of Zurich
Plattenstrasse 11
8032 Zurich
Switzerland
daniel.thoma@zzm.uzh.ch

Pietro Venezia
DDS
Adjunct Professor
Department of Prosthodontics
University of Catania (Italy)
and
Private practice
Via G. Posca, 15
70124 Bari (BA)
Italy
pierovenezia@gmail.com

Table of Contents

1 <u>Introduction</u>

M. Roccuzzo

In the earlier days of implant dentistry, osseointegration was considered to be a sufficient condition for long-term successful implant rehabilitation. With time, however, it became evident that soft-tissue integration is of significant importance and that the formation of an early and long-standing effective mucosal barrier, capable of biologically protecting the peri-implant structures, is essential. This soft-tissue barrier is mainly the result of a wound-healing process that results in an effective interface between "living tissues" and a "foreign body" (Rompen and coworkers 2006).

Whether the presence of a minimum amount of keratinized mucosal (KM) is necessary for the long-term maintenance of peri-implant health has been controversial for many years. Several researchers have found that insufficient KM may be correlated with plaque accumulation, bleeding on probing, discomfort when brushing, mucosal recession, and peri-implant mucositis (Bouri and coworkers 2008; Boynueğri and coworkers 2013; Chung and coworkers 2006; Roccuzzo and coworkers 2016). Other researchers were unable to obtain similar findings (Frisch and coworkers 2015), with some even suggesting that KM may not be essential in the presence of scrupulous oral hygiene and rigorous compliance with a professional maintenance regimen (Lim and coworkers 2019).

On the other hand, complete osseointegration and perfect soft-tissue integration are not necessarily correlated with successful esthetic rehabilitation of a missing tooth or teeth. Indeed, success criteria for esthetically sensitive areas must include measurements of the peri-implant mucosa, as well as the restoration and its relationship to the surrounding dentition (Belser and coworkers 2004).

Apart from the prosthetic aspects, sufficient horizontal and vertical volume is also essential for long-term esthetic soft-tissue stability. Where soft-tissue deficiencies exist, appropriate augmentation procedures may be required for comprehensive rehabilitation. Recent advances in implant dentistry have provided clinicians with various treatment options to treat peri-implant soft-tissue defects. At the same time, though, soft-tissue grafting procedures are of moderate to high complexity and may be associated with a significant risk of complications. For this reason, various step-by-step procedures have been outlined and illustrated by individual case descriptions for the reader of this book.

The aim of this ITI Treatment Guide is to foster awareness of the increasing demands on clinicians to provide treatment for a growing population of patients with soft-tissue related problems. The authors hope that Volume 12 will be a valuable resource and reference work for the treatment of patients with mucogingival deformities to reduce the risk of biological and esthetic complications and to ensure predictable and stable long-term results.

2 Importance of the Peri-Implant Soft Tissues

A. Sculean

Dental implants are anchored in jawbone via direct contact between the bone and the implant, a phenomenon called *osseointegration* (Albrektsson and coworkers 1981). Emerging evidence indicates that the long-term success and survival of implants does not depend solely on osseointegration, but also on the soft tissues around the transmucosal aspect of the implant that separate the peri-implant bone from the oral cavity. This soft-tissue seal or collar is also called the *peri-implant mucosa* (Lindhe and coworkers 2008). The attachment of the soft tissue to the implant serves as a biological seal that ensures healthy conditions and prevents the development of peri-implant infections (peri-implant mucositis and peri-implantitis). Consequently, the peri-implant soft tissues play a crucial role for long-term implant survival (Lindhe and coworkers 2008).

The soft tissue around teeth develops during tooth eruption and seals the supporting tissues (the alveolar bone, periodontal ligament, and cementum) against the oral cavity (Bosshardt and Lang 2005). The peri-implant mucosa forms after traumatizing the oral soft and hard tissues to accommodate osseointegrated implants. The following presents a brief description of the most important anatomical features of the periodontal and peri-implant tissues.

Structure of periodontal tissues in health

The periodontium comprises the tissues supporting the teeth: the tooth-facing part of the *gingiva*, the *root cementum*, the *periodontal ligament*, and the part of the alveolar process that lines the tooth socket, termed *alveolar bone* (Schroeder and Listgarten 1997) (Figs 1 to 5).

As they develop, the teeth penetrate the epithelial lining of the oral cavity and then persist as transmucosal organs. Their root portion is anchored in the bone, while the crown resides in the oral cavity. The most important function of the gingiva is to protect the underlying soft and hard connective tissues from penetration by microorganisms from the oral cavity. The gingiva terminates coronally at the gingival margin; apically it ends at the mucogingival junction or becomes continuous with the mucosa of the hard palate. The gingival sulcus has an

approximate depth of 0.5 mm; however, in a completely healthy situation, it may not be clinically detectable (Schroeder and Listgarten 1997).

The interdental region contains a structure called the *gingival papilla*. The gingiva consists of two parts, the *free gingiva* and the *attached gingiva*. The free gingiva comprises the coronal portion of the gingiva and follows the contour of the cementoenamel junction, varying in width between 1 and 2 mm (Ainamo and Löe 1966). Its apical boundary is accentuated by a stippled line; a gingival groove may also be present. The attached gingiva stretches between the end of the free gingiva and the alveolar mucosa, or the mucosa of the floor of the mouth. Because the palatal mucosa extends to the free gingiva, there is no attached gingiva in the palate. The width of the attached gingiva may range from 1 to 10 mm (Ainamo and Löe 1966).

Junctional epithelium

The *junctional epithelium* is a non-keratinized epithelium that, due to its unique structural and functional adaptation, plays a critical role in maintaining periodontal health by providing a functional barrier to microbial challenges. Cell division occurs in the basal layer facing the lamina propria, while the innermost cells constitute the *epithelial attachment*. It consists of the basal lamina and hemidesmosomes that connect the epithelial cells with the tooth surface (Bosshardt and Lang 2005).

Connective tissue of the gingiva

The *connective tissue of the gingiva* consists mainly of fibroblasts exhibiting phenotypes that differ from those from the periodontal ligament (Bartold and coworkers 2000). They are arranged as groups of collagen fibers with a complex three-dimensional architecture that allows polymorphonuclear neutrophils (PMNs) and mononuclear cells to migrate through the connective tissue until they can pass the basement membrane bordering the junctional epithelium. Even in clinically healthy circumstances, an inflammatory cell infiltrate will be present and can be considered a common (normal) characteristic of the connective tissue adjacent to the junctional epithelium.

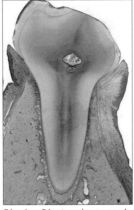

Fig 1 Photomicrograph. Tooth with a healthy periodontium. Supporting tissues of the tooth consisting of the root cementum, periodontal ligament, alveolar bone, and gingiva.

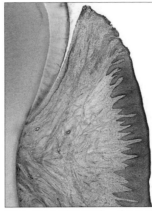

Fig 2 Photomicrograph. Supra-alveolar soft tissue consisting of the oral sulcular epithelium, junctional epithelium, and connective-tissue attachment (collagen fibers inserting into the root cementum). The junctional epithelium ends at the cementoenamel junction (CEJ) at the point of the insertion of the collagen fibers into the root cementum.

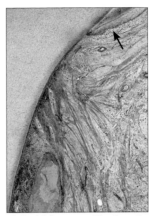

Fig 3 Higher magnification. Supra-alveolar soft tissue comprising the junctional epithelium and root cementum with inserting collagen fibers. Well-encapsulated minor inflammatory cell infiltrate (arrow) located adjacently to the junctional epithelium.

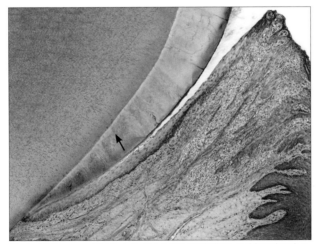

Fig 4 Higher magnification. Oral sulcular epithelium and junctional epithelium. The apical extension of the junctional epithelium ends at the cementoenamel junction. The well-encapsulated inflammatory cell infiltrate (arrow) is clearly distinguishable next to the junctional epithelium.

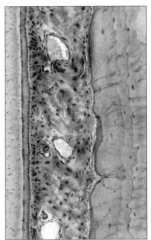

Fig 5 Higher magnification. Intact periodontal ligament connecting the root cementum with the alveolar bone. The collagen fibers invest in both root cementum and alveolar bone.

Periodontal ligament

The soft connective tissue interposed between the alveolar bone and the root cementum is called the *periodontal ligament*. Coronal to the alveolar crest, the periodontal ligament merges with the lamina propria of the gingiva, while it is continuous with the dental pulp periapically. The width of the periodontal ligament measures approximately 200 μm, being thinnest in the middle third of the root. Its width decreases with age.

The most important function of the periodontal ligament is to attach the tooth to the surrounding bone. Another important function is the damping of occlusal forces. Additionally, the periodontal ligament serves as an important reservoir for cells that are constantly needed for tissue homeostasis and play a crucial role in periodontal wound healing and regeneration (periodontal fibroblasts, cementoblasts, odontoclasts, osteoblasts and osteoclasts, epithelial cell rests of Malassez, monocytes and macrophages, and undifferentiated mesenchymal progenitor and stem cells).

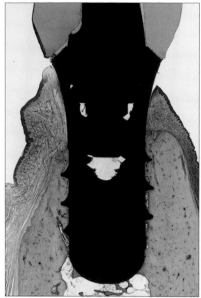

Fig 6   Photomicrograph. Osseointegrated dental implant with direct bone-to-implant contact and supracrestal soft-tissue implant contact.

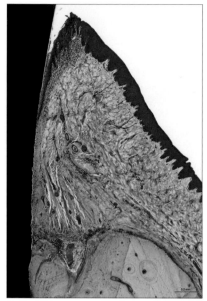

Fig 7   Higher magnification- Supracrestal peri-implant soft tissues consisting of oral and sulcular epithelium and connective tissue adhesion to the implant surface.

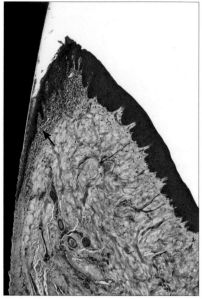

Fig 8   Higher magnification. Coronal portion of the supracrestal peri-implant soft tissues. The oral and sulcular epithelium are clearly visible. The collagen fibers located apically to the junctional epithelium run parallel to the implant surface. A more diffuse inflammatory infiltrate (arrow) is located immediately adjacent the junctional and sulcular epithelium.

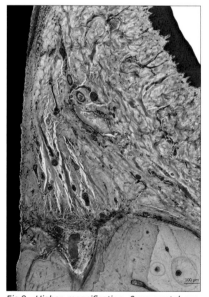

Fig 9   Higher magnification. Supracrestal portion of the peri-implant soft tissues. The collagen fibers located apically to the junctional epithelium run parallel to the implant surface.

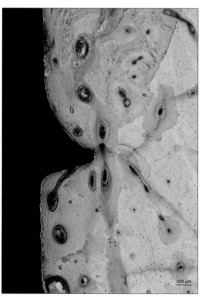

Fig 10   Higher magnification. Direct contact between the bone and the implant surface (osseointegrated implant).

The fibroblasts of the periodontal ligament synthesize, structure, and remodel the extracellular matrix, which consists of collagen fibers and an amorphous ground substance composed of non-collagenous proteins. Due to its structural configuration, the periodontal ligament provides a flexible attachment of the tooth to the surrounding bone via *Sharpey's fibers* into the mineralized tissues (Nanci and Bosshardt 2006).

Root cementum

Root cementum is a mineralized connective tissue coating the roots of teeth, usually extending from the cementoenamel junction to the root apex. Its primary function is to invest and attach the fibers of the periodontal ligament to the root surface (the acellular extrinsic fiber cementum, AEFC, and the cellular mixed stratified cementum, CMSC). However, root cementum also has other important functions, such as adjusting the tooth position to new physiologic requirements and repair of root defects (cellular intrinsic fiber cementum, CIFC) (Nanci and Bosshardt 2006).

Alveolar bone

The teeth are anchored in the *alveolar bone*, a part of the alveolar process that consists of an outer cortical plate, an inner cortical plate, and a central spongiosa. The alveolar process is continuous with the jawbone and can only develop in the presence of teeth. The inner cortical plate lines the alveolus and is also referred to as the alveolar bone.

In fully erupted and periodontally healthy teeth, the contour of the alveolar crest follows the contour of the cementoenamel junction in a coronoapical direction for approximately 2 mm (Saffar and coworkers 1997). The alveolar bone consists of compact bone characterized by the presence of osteons, the structural unit for cortical bone remodeling. The socket wall exhibits many perforations that connect the periodontal ligament with the endosteal or bone-marrow spaces, thus enabling blood and lymph vessels, and nerve fibers, to pass through these openings.

A characteristic component of the alveolar bone is the *bundle bone*, which is deposited in successive layers running parallel to the socket wall. Its typical appearance is determined by the Sharpey's fibers penetrating its layers. The alveolar bone responds to the functional demands placed on it by the processes of resorption and deposition, known as *bone remodeling*.

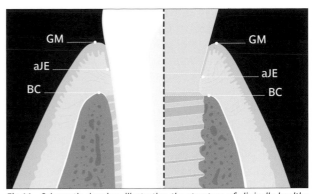

Fig 11   Schematic drawing. illustrating the structure of clinically healthy supra-alveolar soft tissues adjacent to a tooth or an implant (GM: gingival margin, aJE: apical extent of the junctional epithelium, BC: bone crest).

Structure of peri-implant tissues in health

During the process of wound healing following the placement of dental implants, the features of the peri-implant mucosa are established (Sculean and coworkers 2014) (Figs 6 to 10).

Berglundh and coworkers (1991) examined the anatomical and histological features of the peri-implant mucosa in dogs, formed in a two-stage procedure, and compared these with those of the gingiva around teeth. The peri-implant mucosa consisted of a keratinized oral epithelium located at the external surface, connected to a thin barrier epithelium facing the abutment (the equivalent to the junctional epithelium around teeth), the *peri-implant junctional epithelium*. It terminated 2 mm apical to the coronal soft-tissue margin and 1.0 to 1.5 mm coronal to the peri-implant bone crest. The mean supracrestal soft tissue (including the sulcus depth) measured 3.80 mm around implants and 3.17 mm around teeth. While there was no statistically significant difference in the height of the junctional epithelium and sulcus depth between implants and teeth, the height of the soft connective tissue was statistically significantly greater around implants than around teeth (Fig 11).

The peri-implant junctional epithelium and the soft connective tissue adjacent to the abutment appeared to be in direct contact with the implant/abutment surface (Berglundh and coworkers 1991). In summary, the findings of this study showed that the peri-implant mucosa displays comparable anatomical features to those of gingiva around teeth (Berglundh and coworkers 1991).

Subsequent studies provided evidence that a similar mucosal attachment is formed on titanium with different implant systems (Buser and coworkers 1992; Abrahamson and coworkers 1996) and around implants placed using both non-submerged and submerged approaches (Abrahamson and coworkers 1999; Arvidson and coworkers 1996; Weber and coworkers 1996). However, the peri-implant junctional epithelium was significantly longer in implants placed using a submerged approach, where an abutment was connected in a second-stage surgical procedure, than in implants placed using a non-submerged approach (Weber and coworkers 1996).

The *biologic width* (of the supracrestal soft tissue) was revisited in a further dog experiment, following connection of the abutment to the implant with or without a reduced vertical dimension of the oral mucosa (Berglundh and coworkers 1996). It was found that while the peri-implant junctional epithelium was about 2 mm in depth, the supra-alveolar soft connective compartment had a depth of approximately 1.3 to 1.8 mm.

Interestingly, sites with reduced mucosal thickness consistently revealed marginal bone resorption, thus adjusting the width of the supracrestal soft tissue. Evaluating the biologic width around one- and two-piece titanium implants placed in a non-submerged or submerged approach in the mandibles of dogs, Hermann and coworkers (2001) suggested that the gingival margin is located coronally and the biologic width is more similar to teeth around one-piece non-submerged implants than either two-piece non-submerged or two-piece submerged implants. These findings were later confirmed in a comparably designed dog study with another implant system (Pontes and coworkers 2008).

Several studies evaluated the impact of surface topography (surface roughness measurements) on the peri-implant mucosa. Cochran and coworkers (1997) failed to show any differences in the dimensions of the sulcus depth, peri-implant junctional epithelium, and soft connective tissue in contact with implants with a titanium plasma-sprayed (TPS) surface or a sandblasted and acid-etched surface. Abrahamsson and coworkers (2001, 2002) observed similar epithelial and soft connective tissue components on rough (acid etched) and smooth (turned) titanium surfaces. The biologic width (supracrestal soft tissue) was greater on the rough surfaces, although with no statistically significant difference to that around smooth surfaces.

Findings from two human histologic studies revealed less epithelial downgrowth and a longer soft connective tissue compartment in conjunction with oxidized or acid-etched titanium compared to a machined surface (Glauser and coworkers 2005; Ferreira Borges and Dragoo 2010). In a study in baboons, Watzak and coworkers (2006) showed that implant surface modifications had no significant effect on the biologic width after eighteen months of functional loading. Following a healing period of three months, nanoporous TiO_2 coatings of one-piece titanium implants showed similar length of peri-implant soft connective tissue and epithelium than the uncoated, smooth neck portion of the control titanium implants in dogs (Rossi and coworkers 2008). Schwarz and coworkers (2007) have suggested that soft-tissue integration was more influenced by hydrophilicity than by microtopography.

A number of studies revealed that epithelial cells attach to different implant materials in a comparable manner to that in which junctional epithelial cells attach to the tooth surface via hemidesmosomes and a basal lamina (Sculean and coworkers 2014).

Analyzing the intact interface between soft connective tissue and titanium-coated epoxy resin implants, Listgarten confirmed the parallel orientation of collagen fibers to the titanium layer (Listgarten and coworkers 1992, 1996). Since implants lack a cementum layer into which the peri-implant collagen fibers can invest, the attachment of the soft connective tissue to the transmucosal portion of an implant is regarded as being weaker than the soft connective tissue attachment to the surface of a tooth root (Sculean and coworkers 2014). Therefore, improving the quality of the soft tissue-implant interface is of great relevance for maintaining healthy peri-implant tissues (Sculean and coworkers 2014).

The wound-healing sequence leading to the establishment of the soft tissue seal at implants was evaluated by Berglundh and coworkers (2007). Immediately after implant placement, a coagulum occupied the implant-mucosa interface. Numerous neutrophils infiltrated the blood clot, and at four days an initial mucosal seal was established. In the next few days, the number and distribution of leukocytes decreased, becoming confined to the coronal portion, with fibroblasts and collagen dominating the apical part of the implant-tissue interface.

Between one and two weeks of healing, the peri-implant junctional epithelium was located approximately 0.5 mm apical to the mucosal margin. At two weeks, the peri-implant junctional epithelium began to proliferate in an apical direction. After two weeks, the peri-implant mucosa was rich in cells and blood vessels. At four weeks of healing, the peri-implant junctional epithelium migrated further apically and occupied 40% of the total soft-tissue/implant interface. This soft connective tissue was rich in collagen and fibroblasts and was well-organized.

The apical migration of the peri-implant junctional epithelium was completed between six and eight weeks, and the fibroblasts formed a dense layer over the titanium surface at that time. From six to twelve weeks, maturation of the soft connective tissue had occurred; the peri-implant junctional epithelium occupied about 60% of the entire implant/soft-tissue interface. Further away from the implant surface, the number of blood vessels was low; fibroblasts were located between thin collagen fibers, running mainly parallel to the implant surface.

These findings indicate that the soft-tissue attachment to transmucosal (non-submerged) implants made of commercially pure titanium with a polished surface in the neck portion requires at least six weeks (Berglundh and coworkers 2007). These findings from animal experiments were corroborated in human studies by Tomasi and coworkers (2013), indicating that a soft-tissue barrier adjacent to titanium implants may form completely within eight weeks. Further studies have provided evidence indicating that in dogs, the dimensions of the soft-tissue seal (the biologic width or supracrestal soft tissue) around implants are stable for at least twelve (Cochran and coworkers 1997; Assenza and coworkers 2003) or fifteen months, respectively (Hermann and coworkers 2000).

The role of keratinized mucosa in maintaining peri-implant tissue health

It is generally accepted that the assessment of peri-implant health is based on clinical and radiographic parameters bleeding on probing (BOP), probing depth (PD), and marginal peri-implant bone level (Salvi and coworkers 2012; Jepsen and coworkers 2015).

The influence of the presence or absence and the thickness of keratinized or attached mucosa (KAM) on peri-implant tissue health and stability is controversial (Bengazi and coworkers 1996; Schou and coworkers 1992; Strub and coworkers 1991; Wennström and coworkers 1994).

On one hand, a number of clinical studies have failed to show a correlation between the presence of an "adequate" band (2 mm or more) of KAM and implant stability, as assessed by peri-implant bone level or probing depths (Bengazi and coworkers 1996; Wennström and coworkers 1994; Chung and coworkers 2006; Bouri and coworkers 2008; Boynueğri and coworkers 2013). These results were also supported by findings from an animal study indicating that the presence of an "adequate" width of KAM does not significantly influence peri-implant tissue conditions (Strub and coworkers 1991).

However, other clinical studies have suggested that an inadequate (2 mm or less) width of KAM is related to a higher risk of peri-implant inflammation and loss of soft and hard tissue (Warrer and coworkers 1995; Block and coworkers 1996; Zarb and coworkers 1990). A number of other studies have reported statistically significant associations between a peri-implant KAM width of less than 2 mm and higher bleeding scores (Zigdon and coworkers 2008; Adibrad and coworkers 2009; Schrott and coworkers 2009; Lin and coworkers 2013), greater plaque accumulation (Chung and coworkers 2006: Bouri and coworkers 2008; Boynueğri and coworkers 2013; Adibrad and coworkers 2009; Schrott and coworkers 2009; Crespi and coworkers 2010), and more mucosal inflammation (Chung and coworkers 2006; Bouri and coworkers 2008; Boynueğri and coworkers 2013; Adibrad and coworkers 2009; Crespi and coworkers 2010), compared to sites with adequate KAM width (2 mm or more).

3 Soft-Tissue Management Around Tissue-Level Implants

M. Roccuzzo

3.1 Soft-Tissue Management at Implant Placement

From the biological point of view, the apicocoronal positioning of an implant, particularly those of tissue-level design, should follow the principle of "as shallow as possible, as deep as necessary" (Buser and coworkers 2004) in order to avoid deep peri-implant probing depths, taking into account the prosthetic and esthetic factors in the area.

This concept has recently been confirmed in a case-control study on 19 patients that evaluated the modifying effect of a deep mucosal tunnel (DMT, $\geq$ 3 mm) on the induction and resolution phases of experimental peri-implant mucositis (Chan and coworkers 2019). All patients, each with a properly placed tissue-level implant, were assigned either to the test group (DMT, depth $\geq$ 3 mm) or to the control group (shallow mucosal tunnel, SMT, $\leq$ 1 mm). The subjects underwent a standard experimental peri-implant mucositis protocol, characterized by an oral-hygiene optimization phase, a three-week induction phase using an acrylic stent to prevent self-performed oral hygiene at the experimental implant, and a three-plus-two-week resolution phase.

The modified plaque index (mPI), gingival index (mGI), and IL-1β concentrations in the peri-implant sulcus fluid were determined over time. Both the mPI and the mGI increased during the induction phase. After normal oral hygiene had resumed, the mPI and mGI resolved towards baseline values in the SMT group, while they diverged in the DMT group. Although plaque accumulation was resolved in the DMT group, the resolution of inflammation was delayed and found to be of smaller magnitude during the first three weeks after resumption of oral hygiene. IL-1β Concentrations were significantly higher in the DMT group at the end of induction and during the resolution phase, corroborating the clinical findings. Removal of the crown and submucosal professional cleaning were needed to revert mGI to baseline values in the DMT group.

The fact that the depth of the peri-implant sulcus influenced the resolution of experimental mucositis raised doubts as to the efficacy of self-performed oral hygiene in scenarios where implants are placed too deeply. Therefore, since the risk of mucositis evolving into peri-implantitis appears to be higher in such clinical situations, clinicians should make every effort to place implants properly—not only for esthetic, but also for biological reasons (Berglundh and coworkers 2018).

It should be noted that, from a clinical point of view, this may be more easily achievable for implants without adjacent teeth, but more challenging if the implant has to be placed between two teeth, particularly if these teeth are periodontally compromised. Figures 1a-b show examples of correct implant positioning. Figures 2a-b show examples of incorrect implant positioning.

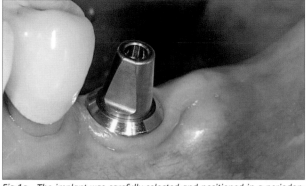

Fig 1a   The implant was carefully selected and positioned in a periodontally compromised patient so as to present minimal probing depth (time of crown cementation).

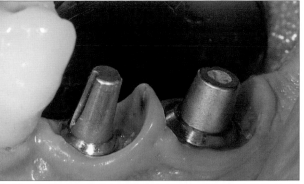

Fig 1b   Healthy interdental papilla between two tissue-level implants, after removing seven-year-old single ceramic crowns which had been kept in place with provisional cement.

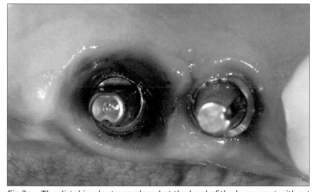

Fig 2a   The distal implant was placed at the level of the bone crest without considering the thickness of the soft tissue, resulting in a deep mucosal tunnel.

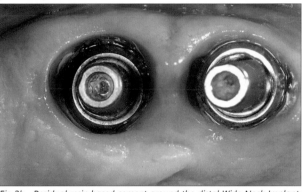

Fig 2b   Residual resin-based cement around the distal Wide Neck Implant. The deep mucosal tunnel does not allow complete removal of the excess cement. Screw-retained restorations would have been preferable in both cases.

The ideal implant position for optimal soft-tissue integration should be planned before removing the teeth. Ridge preservation is one of the treatment options after tooth extraction, particularly in situations where one or more socket walls are missing (Roccuzzo and coworkers 2014c; Mardas and coworkers 2015). The rationale for this approach is that the maintenance of the ridge contour often facilitates subsequent treatment steps and limits the risk of an improper position of the implant collar, creating an ideal soft-tissue seal (MacBeth and coworkers 2017). Figures 3a-i show an example of long-term soft-tissue stability after implant placement following ridge preservation. The correct positioning of an implant, with a shallow peri-implant sulcus, could be particularly difficult in areas where the mucosa is too thick. Here an appropriate flap design is mandatory, especially if cemented restorations are planned. Figures 4a-h show an example of implant positioning in the posterior maxilla where a tissue excess needed to be removed.

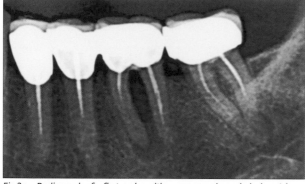

Fig 3a   Radiograph of a first molar with a severe endo-perio lesion. A large post-extraction bone defect with reduced bone levels near the adjacent teeth was anticipated, and therefore ridge preservation was planned.

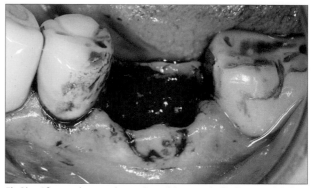

Fig 3b   After tooth extraction and careful removal of inflamed epithelium around the socket border, the marginal mucosa appeared mobile due to the lack of buccal bone.

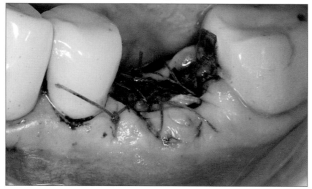

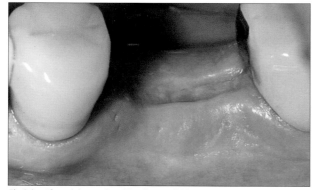

Fig 3c   Deproteinized bovine bone mineral (DBBM) with 10% collagen (Bio-Oss Collagen; Geistlich, Wolhusen, Switzerland) was inserted to fill the decontaminated socket and covered with a double layer of collagen membrane (Bio-Gide; Geistlich) secured with 4-0 Vicryl (Ethicon; Johnson & Johnson International) resorbable sutures.

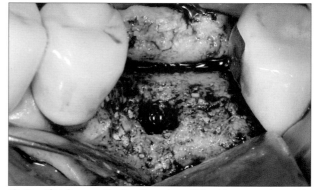

Fig 3d   After eight weeks of healing, a thick band of keratinized mucosa was visible.

Fig 3e   After four months, the dimensions of the ridge were adequate to insert a fixture in the proper position, with no need for further augmentation.

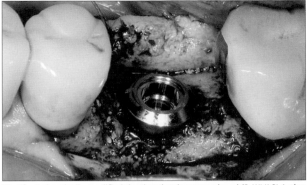

Fig 3f   A chemically modified titanium implant was placed (S, WNI SLActive, diameter 4.8 mm, length 12 mm; Institut Straumann AG, Basel, Switzerland).

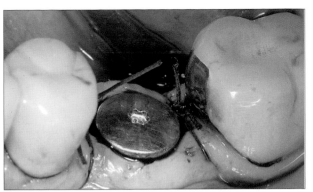

Fig 3g   The soft tissues were circumferentially adapted around the smooth collar of the implant for ideal non- submerged suturing.

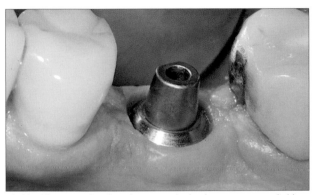

Fig 3h   Three months after placement, the implant was surrounded by a firm collar of keratinized tissue.

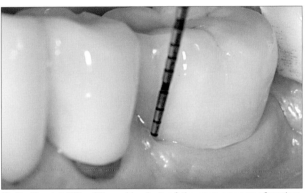

Fig 3i   Good stability of the peri-implant soft tissues seven years after placement despite some buccal recession on the adjacent natural premolar.

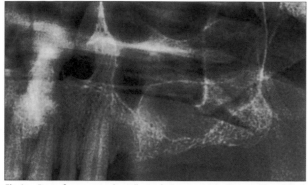

Fig 4a   Part of a panoramic radiograph. Large cyst in the maxillary left sinus. After consultation with an ENT surgeon, who did not suggest any specific treatment, it was decided to place implants without interfering with the sinus.

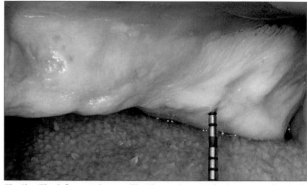

Fig 4b   The left posterior maxilla. The probe used for bone sounding indicated the presence of very thick mucosa in the area of the second molar.

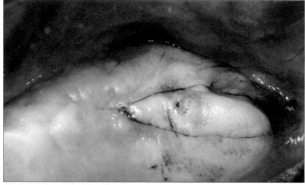

Fig 4c   Primary incision lines.

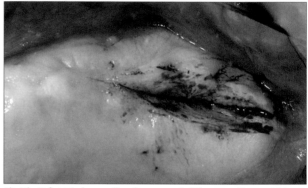

Fig 4d   Left posterior maxilla after removal of the excess tissue, which was later used as a graft in the anterior area.

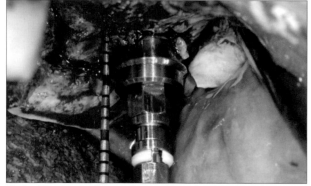

Fig 4e   Titanium implant at site 27 with a chemically modified surface (S, WNI SLActive, diameter 4.8 mm, length 10 mm; Institut Straumann AG). The standard implant with a 2.8-mm smooth collar was considered ideal for bringing the margin of the restoration to a more coronal level.

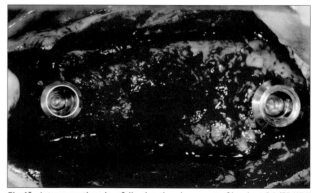

Fig 4f   Intraoperative view following the placement of implant 24 (SP, WNI SLActive, diameter 4.1 mm, length 12 mm; Institut Straumann AG). The implant with a 1.8-mm collar was selected to reduce the risk of future soft-tissue dehiscences. The bone concavity on the buccal aspect of the mesial implant is a risk factor for dehiscence.

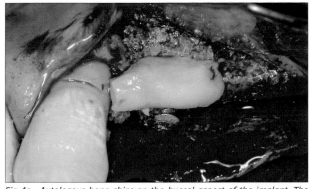

Fig 4g Autologous bone chips on the buccal aspect of the implant. The connective-tissue graft taken from the posterior area was adapted to protect the bone chips and to increase the width of the crest.

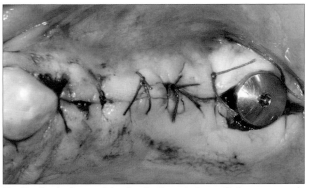

Fig 4h Semi-submerged healing in the anterior grafted area; non-submerged healing with close adaptation of the flap around the collar of the distal implant.

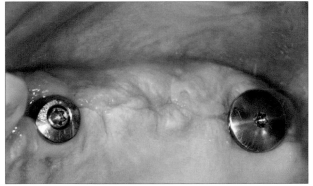

Fig 4i Optimal adaptation of the soft tissues around both implants six weeks after implant placement.

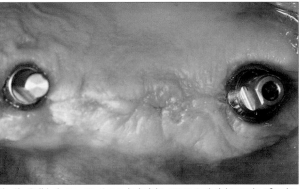

Fig 4j Solid abutments, 4 mm in height, connected eight weeks after implant placement.

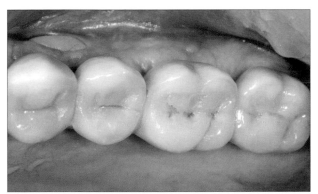

Fig 4k Four-unit cemented metal-ceramic bridge in situ.

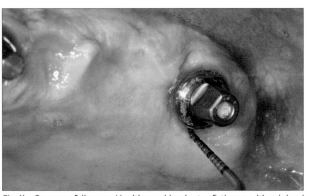

Fig 4l One-year follow up. Healthy peri-implant soft tissues with minimal probing depth (< 4 mm) and no bleeding after removing the provisionally cemented ceramic bridge.

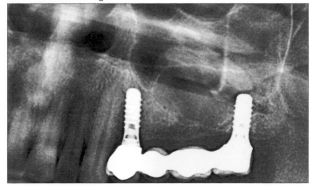

Fig 4m Radiograph at the five-year follow-up. Stable interproximal bone levels.

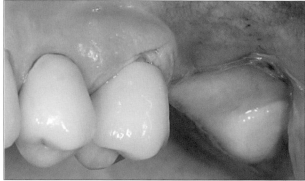

Fig 5a   *Preoperative situation.*

One of the challenges in optimal flap design around non-submerged implants is the circumferential closure around the implant collar, especially when the soft tissues present anatomical irregularities. Figures 5a-k show an example of soft-tissue management for non-submerged tissue-level implants in the posterior maxilla with an irregular soft-tissue morphology.

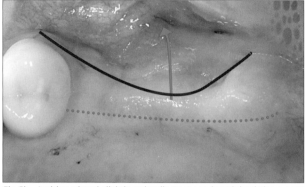

Fig 5b   *Incision placed slightly palatally to move keratinized tissue onto the buccal side.*

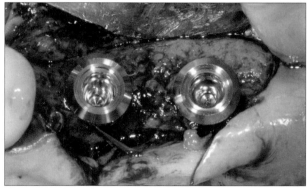

Fig 5c   *Two wide-neck implants placed at sites 26 and 27 (SP, WNI SLActive, diameter 4.8 mm, length 10 mm; Institut Straumann AG).*

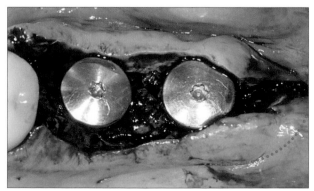

Fig 5d   *Incision on the distal portion of the palatal flap.*

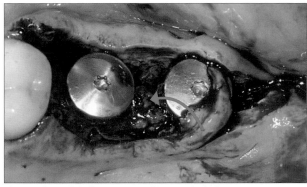

Fig 5e   The pedicle flap was rotated counterclockwise.

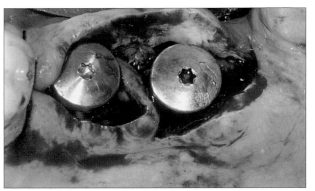

Fig 5f   Pedicle inserted between the two implants.

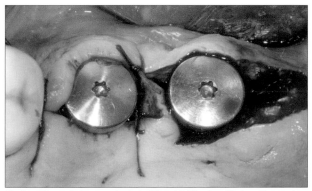

Fig 5g   The pedicle was adapted with a 4-0 Vicryl vertical mattress suture between the 2 implants.

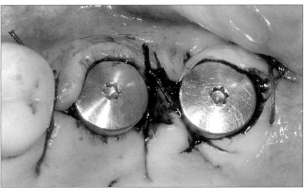

Fig 5h   Final suture, distally to the distal implant.

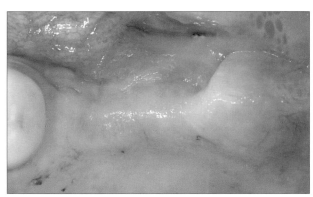

Fig 5i   Preoperative occlusal view.

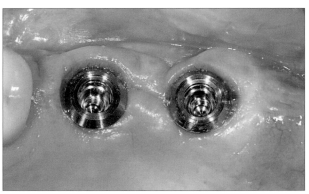

Fig 5j Postoperative occlusal view.

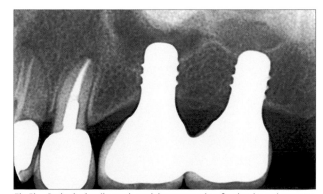

Fig 5k   Periapical radiograph at eighteen months after implant placement. Favorable interproximal bone levels.

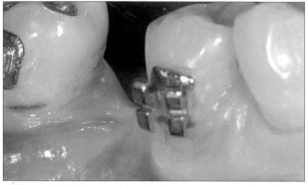

Fig 6a   Preoperative view of site 46, at the end of orthodontic treatment. Limited crestal width and no keratinized mucosa.

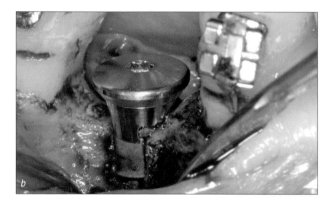

Creating an optimal flap for ideal transmucosal healing becomes even more difficult if no keratinized mucosa is present at all. In these circumstances, a free gingival graft may be advised, especially if bone regeneration is required, as discussed in Chapter 4.1.

Often, a small quantity of keratinized tissue will be sufficient to create a soft-tissue cuff around the implant collar, provided the tissue is properly surgically managed. Figures 6a-l show an example of soft-tissue management around a tissue-level implant in conjunction with bone regeneration in a case where there does not appear to be any keratinized tissue available.

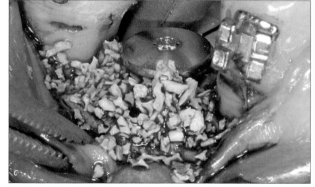

Fig 6b-c   Once the implant was placed (S, SLA, diameter 4.1 mm, length 12 mm; Institut Straumann AG), the dehiscence on the facial bone was covered with autologous bone and a DBBM graft.

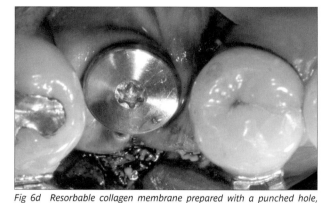

Fig 6d   Resorbable collagen membrane prepared with a punched hole, placed over the graft, and secured with a healing cap.

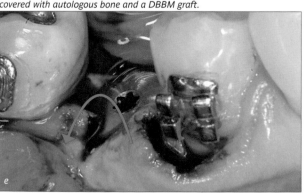

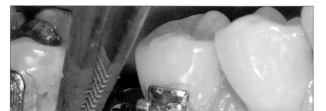

Fig 6e-f   The mesial papilla rotated 90° counterclockwise and sutured to the distal papilla to provide a wide band of keratinized tissue buccally to the implant.

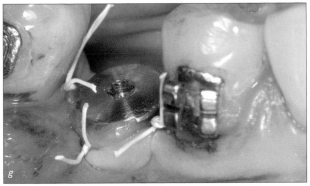
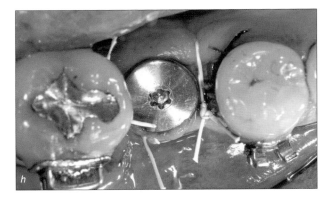

Fig 6g-h   e-PTFE sutures, buccal and occlusal views.

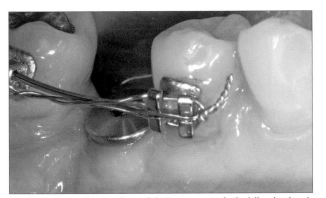
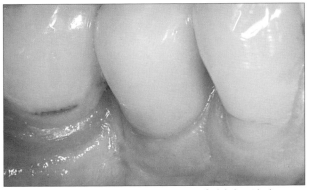

Fig 6i   Early healing (at six weeks). A new mucogingival line is already evident.

Fig 6j   Fifteen months after implant placement, facial view. Ideal contour of the soft tissues thanks to bone grafting and papilla rotation at the time of implant placement.

In many circumstances, poor implant placement may result in restricted access for proper oral hygiene and increase the risk of mucosal inflammation. Plaque accumulation at implant sites causes a more pronounced inflammatory response compared to natural teeth (Berglundh and coworkers 2011). Indeed, even though the evidence is limited, there is a strong common perception that properly placed implants do not present biological complications as frequently as poorly placed implants.

Apart from the prosthetically driven position, a wide band of non-mobile, keratinized mucosa, a correct peri-implant sulcus, and a thick tissue phenotype might seem desirable, if not essential, for reducing the incidence of tissue inflammation and long-term complications around implants.

3.2   Soft-Tissue Management Before Implant Placement

On the occasion of the 2017 World Workshop, Hämmerle and Tarnow (2018) reported that a significant amount of controlled prospective studies with medium-size patient samples indicated that thin soft tissue around implants leads to increased peri-implant marginal bone loss compared to thick soft tissue. Most of the data, however, were published by one group of researchers.

Linkevicius and coworkers (2009) placed 46 implants in 19 patients. The implants were divided into two groups related to soft-tissue thickness. At the one-year follow-up, the marginal bone loss at the implants in the thin-tissue group was on the order of 1.5 mm, compared to only 0.3 mm in the thick-tissue group.

In addition, the same investigators analyzed the effects of buccal soft-tissue thickness on marginal bone-level changes in 32 patients. They found a significant correlation between soft-tissue thickness and bone loss, with thin soft-tissue sites presenting more bone loss (0.3 mm versus 0.1 mm) at the one-year follow-up.

That thin soft tissue leads to increased marginal bone loss was confirmed in another recent study (Linkevicius and coworkers 2015). In addition to the thin-tissue and thick-tissue groups, the investigators followed a third group of about 30 patients whose thin soft tissue was augmented by grafting at the time of implant. The resulting bone loss was not different from that in thick soft-tissue group. These findings seem to indicate that adequate soft-tissue thickness benefits the stability of the peri-implant bone levels.

In another study, Puisys and Linkevicius (2015) concluded that, since significantly less bone loss can occur in naturally thick soft tissue than in patients with a thin tissue phenotype, augmenting the tissue could be the way to reduce crestal bone loss.

Based on the observation that significantly less bone loss occurs around implants placed in thick tissue phenotypes compared to thin phenotypes, clinicians may be encouraged to augment thin soft tissue before or during implant placement in order to facilitate crestal bone stability. Figures 7a-i show an example of this treatment approach in the posterior mandible of a 63-year-old woman.

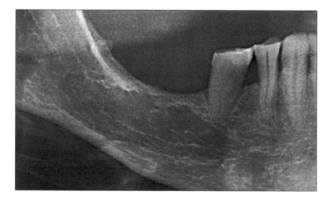

Fig 7a   Panoramic radiograph of the edentulous sites 46 and 47. There is barely enough bone available for implant placement above the mandibular canal.

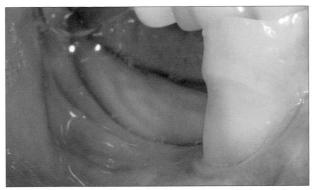

Fig 7b   Edentulous area, buccal view. Very shallow vestibule and absence of keratinized mucosa.

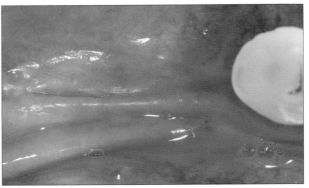

Fig 7c   Edentulous area, occlusal view. Very thin crest.

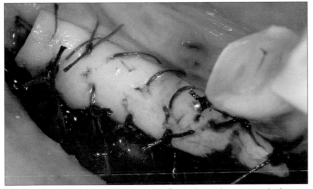

Fig 7d   Free gingival graft harvested from the palate sutured above a split-thickness flap in the area where the implants are planned.

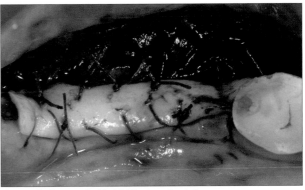

Fig 7e   Graft sutured with 4-0 Vicryl, occlusal view

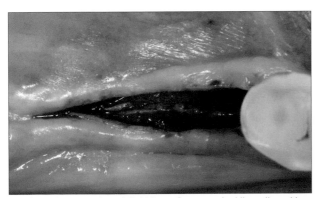

Fig 7f   At three months, a full-thickness flap was raised lingually and buccally for placing the implants. Thicker keratinized tissue on both sides of the flap.

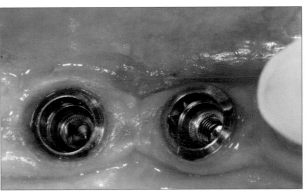

Fig 7g   At the time of the final impression, occlusal view. Both implants are surrounded by a thick collar of keratinized tissue, that creates an effective barrier that protects the peri-implant structures.

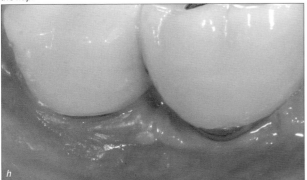

Figs 7h-i   Clinical and radiographic views of the screw-retained ceramic crowns at 6 years. Prosthetic procedures: Dr. Nicola Scotti – Torino, Italy

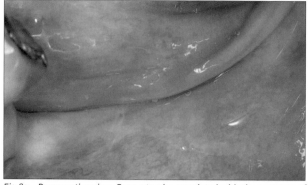

Fig 8a   *Preoperative view. Bone atrophy associated with the presence of very thin mucosa, with almost no keratinization.*

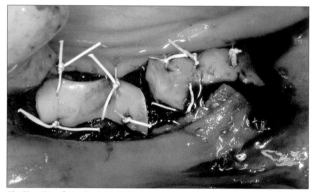

Fig 8b   *Two free gingival grafts sutured in the area where implant placement and bone regeneration was planned.*

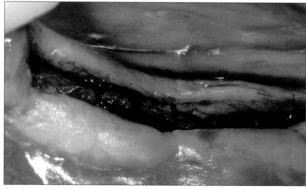

Fig 8c   *Three months after soft-tissue augmentation. A thick band of keratinized tissue was present on the lingual and buccal aspects of the full-thickness flap.*

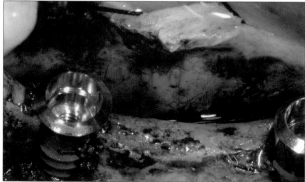

From a clinical perspective, the presence of a wide band of keratinized tissue facilitates the transmucosal healing of dental implants, even in cases where bone regeneration is required, as it allows the creation of a thick soft-tissue cuff around the collar of the implant. Figures 8a-l show an example of this treatment approach in the posterior mandible of a 57-year-old woman, for whom horizontal bone regeneration was needed in conjunction with implant placement.

Several studies have argued the use of various techniques for vertical ridge augmentation in cases of severe atrophy of the alveolar ridge, using either non-resorbable or resorbable membranes supported by a space-making device or a titanium mesh (Esposito and coworkers 2008; Fontana and coworkers 2011; Roccuzzo and coworkers 2017a).

All these studies also showed that the use of a barrier device is a technique-sensitive procedure and subject to surgical complications (Jepsen and coworkers 2019). One of the main reasons for GBR failures is related to exposure of the barrier membrane, leading to bacterial contamination of the surgical area and infection and thereby compromising the regeneration outcome (Sanz and coworkers 2019). Even though there have been no specific studies on this matter, it might be suggested that membrane exposure, especially during the first four weeks postoperatively, may be higher in patients with very thin mucosa, or without keratinization, or with scar tissue. In specific circumstances, it is therefore reasonable to consider optimizing the quantity and quality of the soft tissue before hard-tissue regenerative procedures are carried out.

Fig 8d   *Implants at sites 35 and 37 (S, RN, diameter 3.3 mm, length 10 mm, and S, RN, diameter 4.8 mm, length 10 mm; Institut Straumann AG) with a large dehiscence-type bone defect on the buccal aspect.*

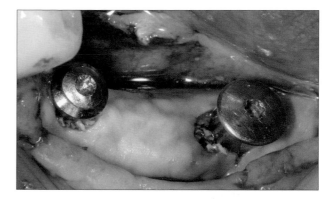

Fig 8e   Guided bone regeneration with autologous bone in contact with the implant surface, followed by a layer of deproteinized bovine bone mineral (DBBM). Resorbable collagen membrane adapted around the implants to stabilize the graft.

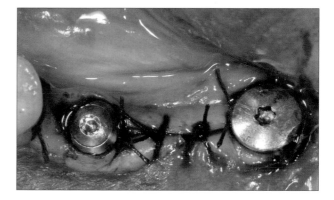

Fig 8f   Sutures for transmucosal healing. Ideal soft-tissue seal around the collar of the implants thanks to the preliminary soft-tissue augmentation.

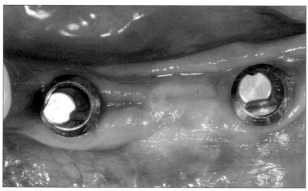

Fig 8g   At the time of delivery of the final prosthesis, occlusal view.

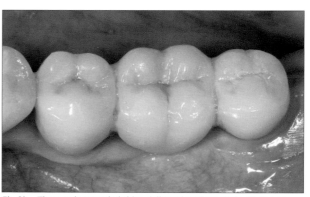

Fig 8h   Three-unit ceramic bridge delivered and secured with temporary cement.

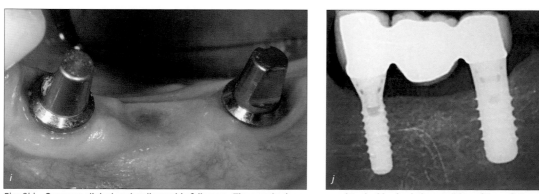

Figs 8i-j   One-year clinical and radiographic follow-up. The prosthesis was removed to double-check the condition of the soft tissues and later then reinserted using definitive cement.

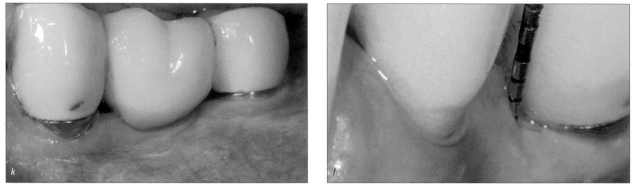

Figs 8k-l   Ten-year follow-up. Minor pigmentation of the ceramic crown on the buccal side. Healthy peri-implant soft tissue with minimal probing depth.

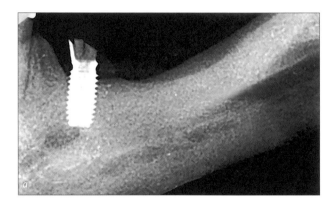

Figures 9a-p exemplify this approach in the mandible of a 63-year-old patient, a dentist and current cigarette smoker. He had previously received an implant at site 35, but it had recently fractured. After surgically removing the fractured implant, vertical bone augmentation was required, as the bone was not high enough to place an implant above the mandibular canal. The examination of the local soft tissue revealed minimal keratinized mucosa and the presence of scar tissue as a result of previous surgery. To reduce the risk of soft-tissue dehiscence and of exposure or infection of the area following GBR, the patient was advised that preliminary soft-tissue augmentation was required prior to any attempt at vertical bone regeneration.

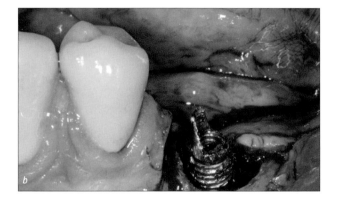

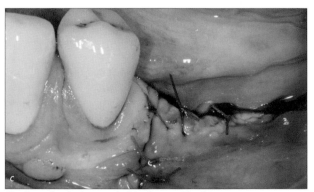

Figs 9a-c   Surgical removal of the fractured implant.

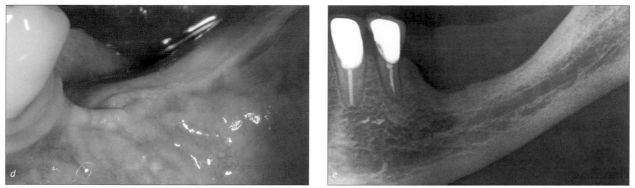

Figs 9d-e   After three months, site 35 presented with minimal keratinized mucosa and scar tissue, considered not to be ideal in view of the planned vertical bone augmentation.

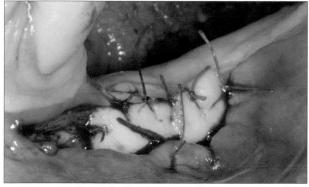

Fig 9f   Free gingival graft sutured on the periosteum after elevating a split-thickness flap, with 4-0 Vicryl.

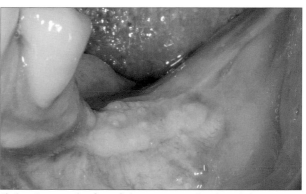

Fig 9g   Four months after soft-tissue augmentation, lateral view.

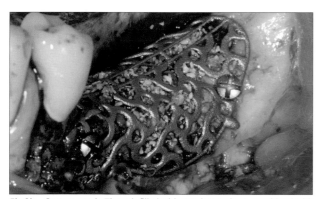

Fig 9h   Custom-made Ti-mesh filled with autologous bone combined with DBBM and secured with two screws to contain and protect the bone graft. The presence of thick mucosa reduced the need for a collagen membrane.

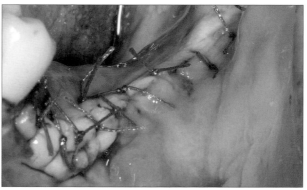

Fig 9i   Flap closed without tension despite coronal advancement and adapted to completely cover the augmented area. The flap was stabilized with Vicryl 3-0 horizontal mattress sutures at the apical aspect and Vicryl 4-0 multiple single interrupted sutures at the far coronal aspect.

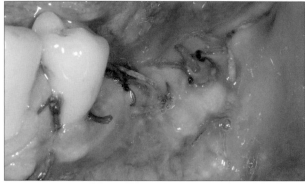

Fig 9j   Two weeks after the surgery. The flap had healed well, and the sutures could be removed.

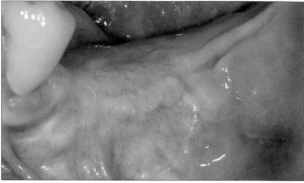

Fig 9k   Clinical view six months after regeneration surgery. Optimal healing.

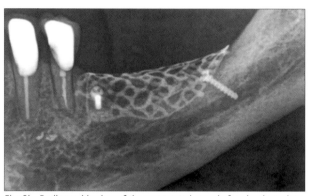

Figs 9l   Radiographic view of the augmented area before implant placement surgery.

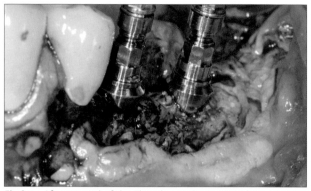

Fig 9m   After removal of the Ti-mesh, two Straumann Tissue Level implants were placed at sites 35 and 36 (SP, RN, diameter 3.3 mm, length 8 mm, and SP, RN, diameter 4.1 mm, length 6 mm; Institut Straumann AG).

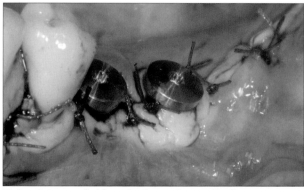

Fig 9n   Sutures applied for optimal non-submerged healing.

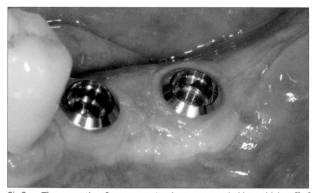

Fig 9o   Three months after surgery. Implants surrounded by a thick cuff of healthy keratinized mucosa. The impressions could now be taken for the final restoration.

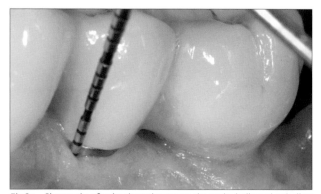

Fig 9p   Six months after implant placement, the probe indicated a shallow sulcus with no signs of inflammation. Prosthetic procedures: Dr. Walter Gino – Torino, Italy

Based on the conclusions of the 2017 World Workshop, namely that a significant amount of controlled prospective studies indicated that thin soft tissue around implants leads to increased marginal bone loss compared to thick soft tissue, clinicians may be encouraged to create ideal soft-tissue conditions before placing implants. Mucogingival surgery may be indicated particularly in patients with thin soft tissue and no keratinization. Each of the two steps of this approach is relatively easy to perform. However, the patient will have to accept the discomfort of two separate interventions not less than a month apart from each other.

Even though recent publications provided guidelines for decision-making if the clinician considers autologous soft-tissue grafting to promote peri-implant health or preserve marginal bone levels at implant sites with insufficient soft-tissue dimensions (Thoma and coworkers 2018a; Giannobile and coworkers 2018), the ideal clinical solution should be individually determined and should represent the results of a proper patient-clinician discussion.

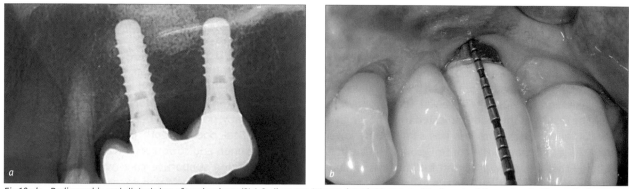

Fig 10a-b   Radiographic and clinical view of two implants (SLA S, diameter 4.1 mm, length 12 mm, and S, diameter 4.1 mm, length 10 mm; Institut Straumann AG), placed two years previously into a thin ridge, presenting with an inferiorly attaching frenulum facially to implant 26. Treatment was indicated to facilitate plaque control and to prevent further progression of the recession.

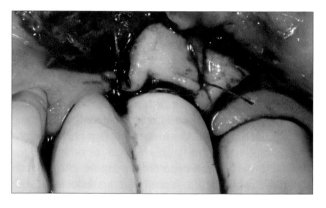
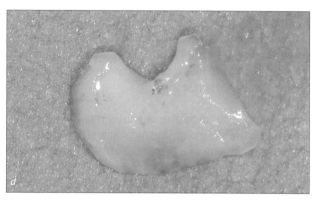

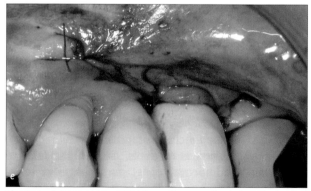
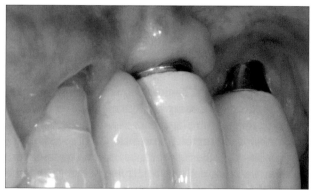

Fig 10c-e   A trapezoidal split-thickness flap was elevated at the implant site. A connective-tissue graft was adapted and placed in a fully submerged approach for optimal blood supply.

Fig 10f   Nine years after the surgical correction. Plaque control was improved around the treated mesial implant, while the soft-tissue dehiscence had increased on the distal implant, which had not received further treatment. The surgical trauma, the shallow vestibule, the lack of keratinized attached mucosa or a thin buccal bone plate at the crestal level may have contributed to the formation of the dehiscence/recession at the most distally located implant.

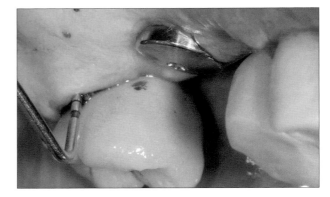

Fig 11a Implant 27, placed nine years previously, palatal view. 13-mm pocket and bleeding on probing. Implant 26 had been placed recently and not yet been loaded. The deep pocket at implant 27 should have been addressed before placing the new implant, or at least at the same time.

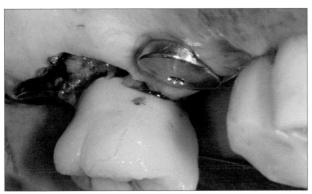

Fig 11b Gingivectomy to eliminate the excessive soft tissue.

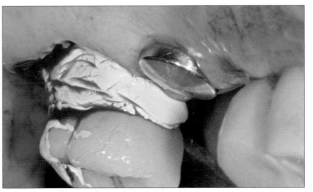

Fig 11c Application of a periodontal dressing.

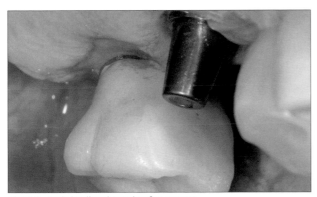

Fig 11d Early healing six weeks after surgery.

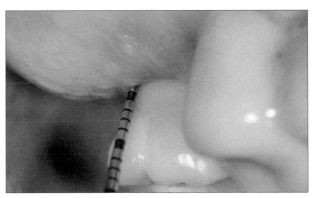

Fig 11e Palatal view of implant 27, presenting with 3-mm probing depth and no bleeding.

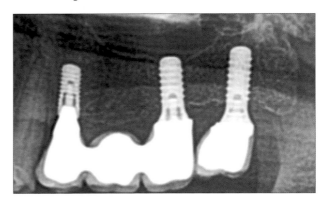

Fig 11f Panoramic radiograph. Ideal peri-implant bone levels around the distal implant at the fifteen-year follow-up.

The main objectives in treating peri-implantitis are:

- decontamination of the implant surface
- removal of infected/inflamed tissue
- creation of a soft-tissue architecture to facilitate oral hygiene.

To achieve this, it is often necessary to elevate a full-thickness flap to remove the granulation tissue resulting from the local inflammation and to decontaminate the implant surface. Depending on the configuration of the defect, a reconstructive approach is often preferred, with or without a membrane. One of the possible negative outcomes of this approach is the creation of a peri-implant soft-tissue dehiscence (Heitz-Mayfield and coworkers 2018a; Roccuzzo and coworkers 2017a). If such a dehiscence raises esthetic concerns, particularly in patients with high esthetic expectations, additional interventions may be required (see Chapter 5.2, Fig 3).

To reduce the need for multiple surgery, particularly if a soft-tissue dehiscence is already present, the surgical treatment of peri-implantitis may be accompanied by the application of a connective-tissue graft (CTG) (Roccuzzo and coworkers 2016). Figures 12a-y illustrate a case where the surgical treatment of a peri-implantitis defect was associated with the application of a CTG.

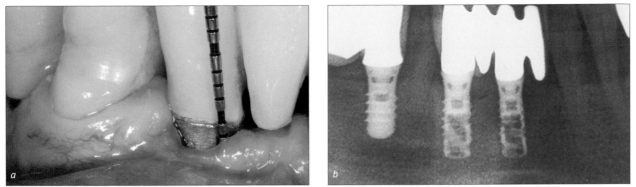

Fig 12a-b   Radiographic and clinical view of a hollow-screw implant placed in November 1994, presenting with a pocket and a soft-tissue dehiscence.

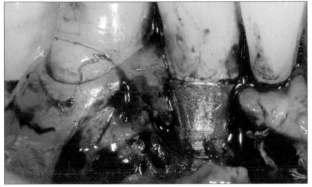

Fig 12c   After raising a full-thickness flap, the granulation tissue was removed with a titanium brush and curettes.

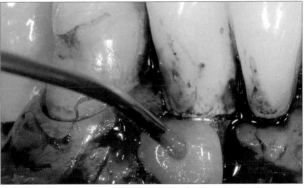

Fig 12d   24% EDTA applied for two minutes for decontamination.

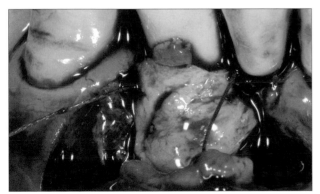

Fig 12e   Connective-tissue graft, taken from the maxillary tuberosity and properly trimmed, adapted over the defect.

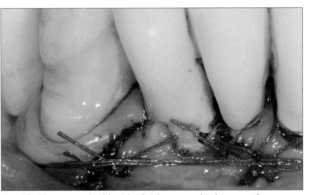

Fig 12f   Flap sutured with 4-0 Vicryl to completely cover the connective-tissue graft.

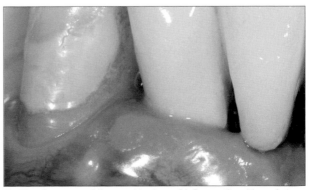

Fig 12g   Seven-year follow-up. No signs of inflammation. The soft-tissue recession was reduced.

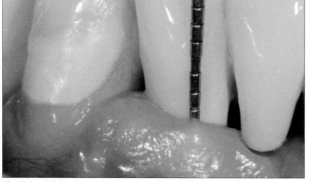

Fig 12 h   Minimal probing depth and no bleeding at the nine-year follow-up visit.

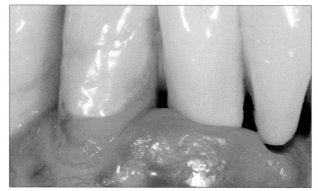

Fig 12 i   Twenty-five years after implant placement. The situation is still stable and free from signs of inflammation.

Recently, a reduced width of keratinized tissue around dental implants has been considered a risk indicator for the severity of peri-implant mucositis (Grischke and coworkers 2019) even in highly compliant, periodontally healthy patients. Based on this observation, in cases of peri-implant mucositis associated with insufficient keratinized tissue, a soft-tissue graft may be indicated to reduce the risk of recurrence. Figures 13a-y illustrate a case where the treatment of severe peri-implant mucositis was accompanied by the application of an FGG graft to improve the quality of the peri-implant soft tissue and to improve the chances of successful long-term maintenance.

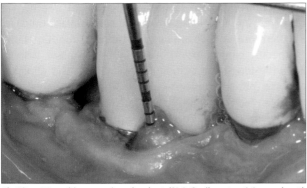

Fig 13a   Mucositis around an implant (SLA S, diameter 4.1 mm, length 8 mm; Institut Straumann AG) placed more than ten years previously.

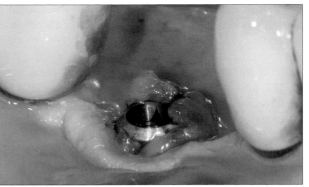

Fig 13b   The crown and abutment were removed to provide access to the inflamed area.

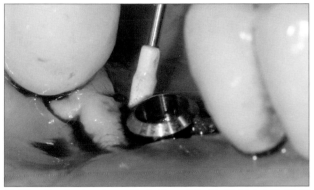

Fig 13c   The treatment consisted of careful debridement and gentle cleaning of the area with titanium curettes and an ultrasonic device with a PTFE-coated tip.

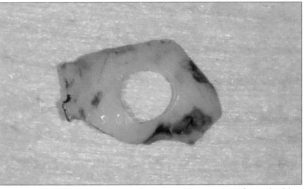

Fig 13d   An FGG was harvested from the palate and perforated with a 4-mm biopsy punch.

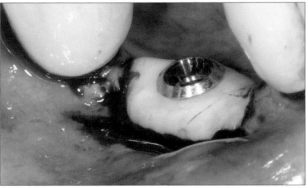

Fig 13e   Precisely adapted FGG around the smooth collar of the implant.

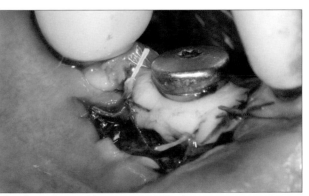

Fig 13f   Graft secured by means of 5-0 Vicryl sutures.

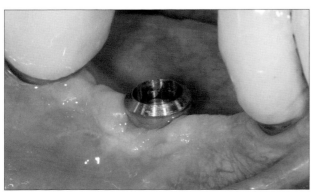

Fig 13g   Six months after treatment.

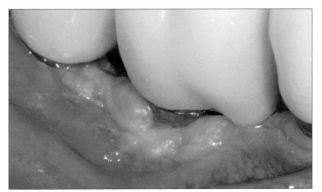

Fig 13 h   New screw-retained ceramic crown in situ.

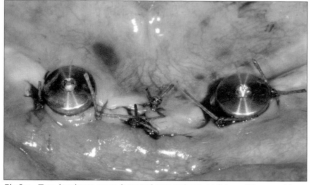

Fig 2a   Two implants were inserted non-submerged in a 66-year-old patient to support an overdenture.

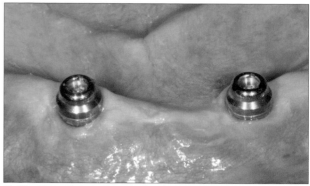

Fig 2b   The patient was instructed to clean properly around each implant; however, he reported discomfort during brushing, particularly on the right-hand side.

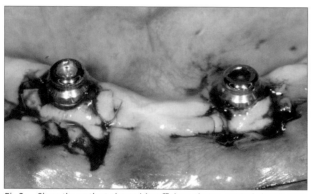

Fig 2c   Since the patient showed insufficient plaque control due to soreness during oral hygiene procedures, he was given the option to receive an additional free gingival graft (FGG) around each implant.

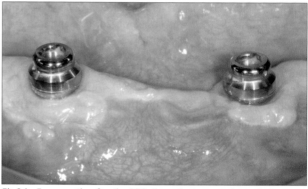

Fig 2d   Four months after the FGG, the patient reported a major improvement in his ability to perform proper plaque control with no discomfort.

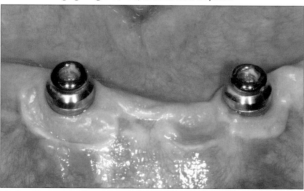

Fig 2e   Two years after the FGG, the mucosa was healthy, with no signs of inflammation and excellent plaque control, even though a small amount of plaque is visible on the inner aspect of the two Locators.

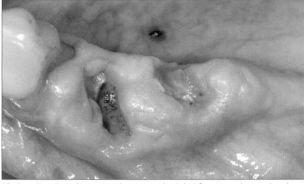

Fig 3a Two hopeless premolar roots scheduled for extraction and replacement with two implants. A type I procedure was selected.

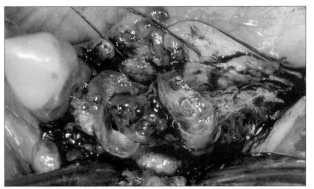

Fig 3b The teeth were carefully extracted.

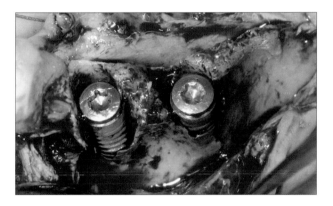

Fig 3c Two submerged implants (BLT, NC SLActive Roxolid, diameter 3.3 mm, length 12 mm; Institut Straumann AG, Basel, Switzerland) were placed at sites 34 and 35 to support a three-unit screw-retained bridge with a distal cantilever.

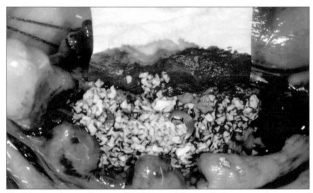

Fig 3d Autologous bone and DBBM particles applied to cover the exposed implant surfaces.

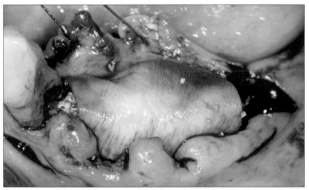

Fig 3e Grafting materials covered with a resorbable collagen membrane.

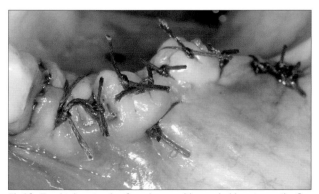

Fig 3f To obtain a tension-free closure with resorbable sutures, the flap needed to be released and stretched, resulting in the mucosa being thinned.

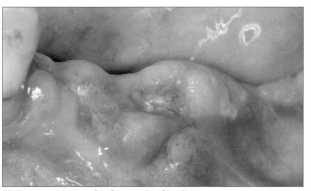

Fig 3g Frontal view after four weeks of healing.

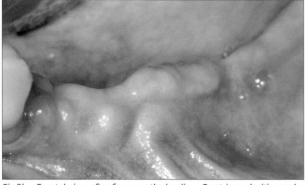

Fig 3h   Frontal view after four months healing. Crest irregularities and a grayish area underneath the stretched alveolar mucosa.

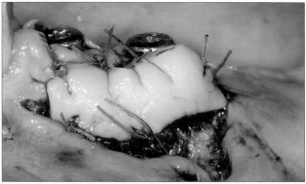

Fig 3i   In conjunction with the second-stage surgery, the depleted residual KM was moved lingually and an FGG was sutured in place buccally on a split-thickness flap.

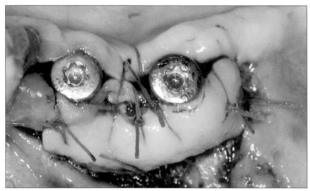

Fig 3j   Occlusal view of the FGG sutured onto the buccal aspect of the two healing caps.

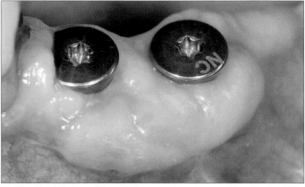

Fig 3k   Frontal view of the soft-tissue contour, two months after the FGG.

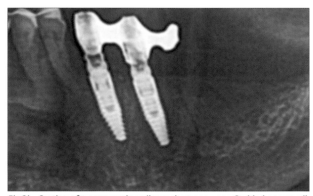

Fig 3l   Section of a panoramic radiograph at one year. Stable bone conditions around both implants.

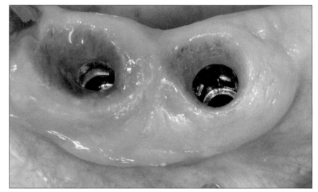

Fig 3 m   Occlusal view of the healthy tissue contours, eighteen months after implant placement. The patient was referred to the prosthodontist for a final impression.

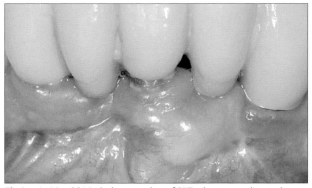

Fig 4a   In May 2014, during a session of SPT, plaque was detected, especially around implant 41 (three years after placement). Motivation, re-instruction, and supragingival instrumentation were performed.

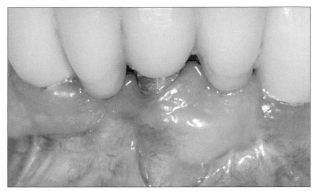

Fig 4b   One year later (May 2015), the overall situation had slightly improved, but an increase in soft-tissue recession can be observed.

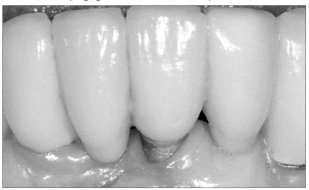

Fig 4c   In November 2017, as the patient still exhibited insufficient plaque control, she was given the option to receive an FGG at the implant to facilitate oral hygiene.

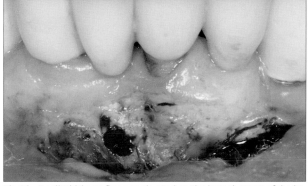

Fig 4d   A split-thickness flap was elevated on the buccal aspect of the implant. Minimal bone dehiscence on the buccal aspect of the area.

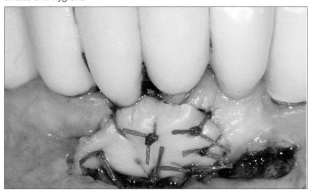

Fig 4e   An FGG is secured by means of resorbable Vicryl sutures.

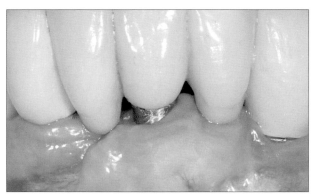

Fig 4f   In July 2019, plaque control had improved.

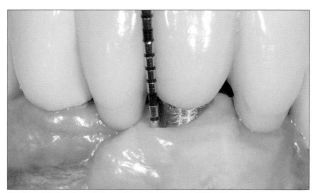

Fig 4g   Minimal pocket depths and absence of bleeding.

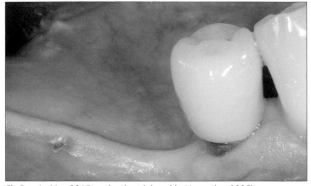

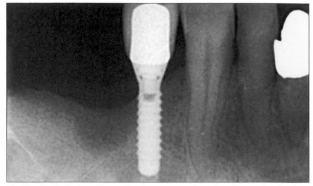

Fig 5a   In May 2015, an implant (placed in November 2006) was supporting the single crown 44. No distal teeth as the patient had recently lost a premolar due to periodontal disease.

Fig 5b   Periapical radiograph. Bone resorption distally to the implant (S, SLA, diameter 3.3 mm, length 10 mm; Institut Straumann AG).

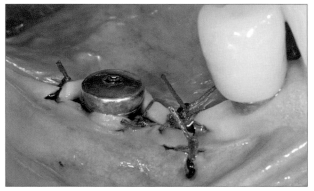

Fig 5c   A non-submerged implant 46 (SP, RNI SLActive, diameter 3.3 mm, length 10 mm, Institut Straumann AG) became the distal support for a three-unit bridge without involving the mucosa around the mesial implant.

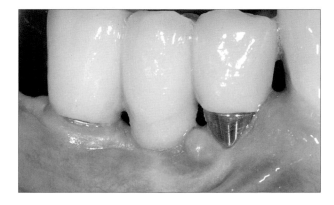

Fig 5d   In June 2016, during a session of supportive periodontal therapy, insufficient plaque control was detected. Furthermore, a progression of the soft-tissue recession was visible around the mesial implant in conjunction with a prominent frenulum. As the rough surface of the implant was almost visible, an FGG was proposed and accepted by the patient.

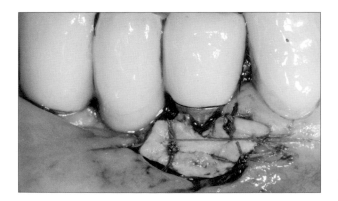

Fig 5e   An FGG was harvested from the tuberosity and sutured after elevating a split-thickness flap.

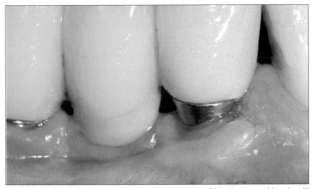

Fig 5f Clinical view at three-years. Plaque control has improved but is still not ideal. A thick cuff of keratinized mucosa is visible around the collar of the mesial implant.

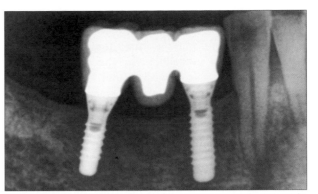

Fig 5g Radiograph demonstrating stable crestal bone levels, even at the distal aspect of the mesial implant placed twelve years previously.

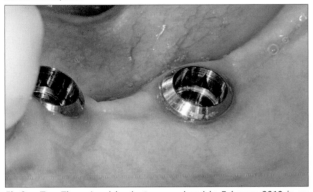

Fig 6a Two Tissue Level implants were placed in February 2010 in an area of the posterior mandible with no keratinized mucosa and a very shallow vestibule.

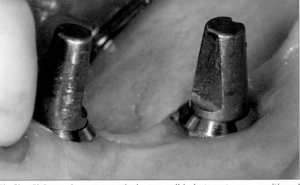

Fig 6b Eight weeks postoperatively, two solid abutments were positioned to support a three-unit bridge.

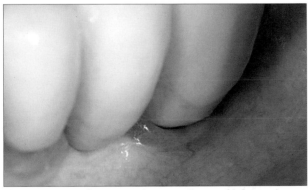

Fig 6c One year after cementation, a small area of inflammation was visible around the collar of the distal implant. An additional intervention to deepen the vestibule with an FGG was decided.

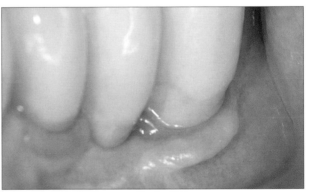

Fig 6d Clinical view, five years after the FGG.

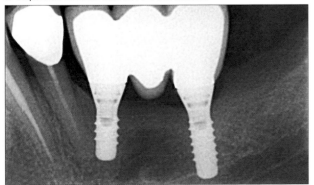

Fig 6e Radiograph at seven years.

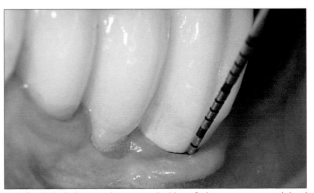

Fig 6f Clinical view at nine years. Stable soft-tissue contours, minimal probing depth, no signs of inflammation, and no recession.

In conclusion, even though there is no definitive consensus regarding the role of KM in preventing biological peri-implant complications, the quoted publications offer preliminary guidelines for the decision-making process. Indeed, it is suggested that KM provides the peri-implant seal with greater resistance to accidental injuries and contributes to the stabilization of the mucosal margin. Apart from potential esthetic advantages, soft-tissue grafting may therefore be indicated wherever there is evidence of mucosal recession or plaque control for the patient is difficult. This might be even more so in erratic/non-compliant maintenance patients, given that by far most patients are not long-term regular compliers in supportive maintenance programs. Reliable mucosal augmentation with an FGG is possible at multiple phases in the course of therapy, and in some circumstances, may be indicated several years after implant placement.

Practitioners considering soft-tissue augmentation should acknowledge and properly discuss the potential complications with the patient, including postoperative discomfort.

It must be mentioned that when an FGG is placed directly over bone, healing will be delayed. Supraperiosteal placement appears to favor better initial adaptation and vascularization of the graft (Dordick and coworkers 1976), with faster healing, as illustrated by the clinical cases presented above. Furthermore, the soft tissue in the tuberosity area is often substantially thicker than at the hard palate, allowing a thick and sufficiently large graft to be harvested with minimal discomfort for the patient (Sanz-Martin and coworkers 2019; Tavelli and coworkers 2019).

Finally, it should be considered that these conclusions are based on the interpretation of the results of the collected studies, albeit with significant heterogeneity in terms of type of patients treated, anatomical regions analyzed, and surgical techniques applied. Therefore, caution and good common sense should always guide the choices of the knowledgeable clinician.

4.2 Soft-Tissue Replacement Materials

A. Sculean

The use of autologous soft-tissue grafts—free gingival grafts (FGG) or connective-tissue grafts (CTG)—has been shown to represent a predictable treatment modality for increasing the width of keratinized attached mucosa (KAM) at dental implants (see Chapter 4.1).

A frequently used technique is the vestibuloplasty (VP), which aims to increase the width of the attached/keratinized mucosa by apically repositioning the soft tissues.

In a randomized controlled clinical study, a total of 64 patients with one implant each presenting a keratinized mucosa width of less than 1.5 mm and showing signs of peri-implant mucositis were treated (Başeğmez and coworkers 2012); 32 implants received free gingival grafts (FGG group) while 32 implants were treated with a vestibuloplasty alone (VP group).

When compared to the use of the vestibuloplasty (VP) alone, the use of FGG resulted in statistically and clinically significantly higher gain in the width of keratinized mucosa than that following VP (2.36 mm in the FGG group versus 1.15 mm in the VP group). Moreover, the use of FGG was associated with a lower postoperative relapse rate than the use of VP alone (2.00 mm in the FGG group versus 3.06 mm in the VP group). This suggested that the application of FGG appears to represent a more predictable method for enhancing the width of the KAM in the vicinity of implants compared with vestibuloplasty alone (Başeğmez and coworkers 2012).

However, despite the positive outcomes reported with the use of autologous soft-tissue grafts, their use is associated with an increase in patient discomfort and pain due to the need for a second surgical site for harvesting donor tissue and potential postoperative complications such as bleeding, numbness, or tissue necrosis at both the donor and recipient sites (Chackartchi and coworkers 2019).

To minimize these shortcomings, efforts have been made in recent decades to develop soft-tissue replacement (grafting) materials that may produce comparable clinical outcomes to those obtained with autologous tissue grafts.

These soft-tissue replacement materials are usually either allogeneic (human-based) or xenogeneic (animal-based).

Acellular dermal allografts
A well-documented soft-tissue replacement graft is the acellular dermal matrix allograft (ADM). Several histological and clinical studies have evaluated its use for various clinical indications, including recession coverage at teeth and a gain of KAM at implants. When ADM was used in conjunction with an apically positioned flap, the graft showed excellent biocompatibility and was filled with new vessels and fibroblasts within the first two weeks after surgery. Epithelialization occurred at six weeks, while complete healing was observed at ten weeks. At six months following surgery, the newly formed tissue had the appearance of a "scar-like" dense connective tissue (Wei and coworkers 2002). However, the findings also indicated that ADM was incapable of influencing/directing the differentiation of the covering epithelium.

In a case series, Park (2006) evaluated the clinical outcomes obtained with ADM to increase the width of the peri-implant keratinized mucosa around implants. A total of 10 patients with an insufficient width of KAM mucosa (2 mm or less) were treated with ADM. At three and six months following treatment, the results revealed an increase in the mean width of the peri-implant keratinized mucosa from 0.8 ± 0.6 mm at baseline to 3.2 ± 0.9 mm at three months and 2.2 ± 0.6 mm at six months, suggesting that ADM appears to be a suitable material for increasing keratinized mucosa width at implants.

In a later study (Başeğmez and coworkers 2013), the use of ADM was compared with that of FGG to increase the width of the peri-implant KAM. Treatment was performed during second stage surgery, before loading the implants. A total of 36 implants were placed in the mandibular central incisor area of 18 patients and subsequently grafted with ADM, while another 18 patients were treated with FGG at 36 implant sites. At six months following surgery, the use of FGG yielded a statistically significantly greater gain of attached mucosa compared to the use of ADM (2.57 mm in the FGG group versus 1.58 mm in the ADM group). Interestingly, ADM showed statistically significantly higher shrinkage compared to FGG (2.68 mm in the ADM group versus 1.73 mm in the FGG group). The results indicate that although the use of ADM allografts may increase the width of peri-implant keratinized mucosa to a certain extent, the use of FGGs seems to yield more predictable outcomes (Başeğmez and coworkers 2013).

Xenogeneic soft-tissue replacement grafts

In the past few decades, various xenogeneic soft-tissue replacement materials (mostly of porcine origin) have been introduced for various clinical indications, such as recession coverage at teeth and gain of keratinized/attached gingiva/mucosa. Histological findings from animal studies and human case reports have demonstrated ingrowth of blood vessels and connective tissue following grafting with xenogeneic materials without any adverse reactions (Vignoletti and coworkers 2014).

Lorenzo and coworkers (2012) compared the use of a xenogeneic collagen matrix of porcine origin with a palatal connective-tissue graft to augment the KAM around implants supporting prosthetic restorations. Six months after grafting, the mean width of KAM was 2.75 ± 1.5 mm at the sites treated with CTG and 2.8 ± 0.4 mm at those treated with collagen matrix, with no statistically significant differences between the two groups. The results also revealed similar esthetic outcomes and a substantial increase in vestibular depth in both groups. The patients treated with the collagen matrix reported less postoperative pain and discomfort than those receiving autologous grafts, although these differences were not statistically significant.

Comparable outcomes in terms of KAM gain were recently also reported by Cairo and coworkers (2017). A total of 60 implants in 60 patients were treated at second-stage surgery with either a collagen matrix or CTG. The results indicated that both procedures resulted in a similar gain in KAM, with no statistically significant differences between treatments. The use of the collagen matrix was associated with statistically significantly less surgical time, less postoperative pain, and greater patient satisfaction than the use of CTG. However, in terms of buccal peri-implant soft-tissue increase, CTG was more effective than the collagen matrix.

In a prospective comparative clinical study, Schmitt and coworkers (2016) compared the long-term outcomes after vestibuloplasty with a porcine collagen matrix to a free gingival graft. A total of 48 patients with atrophic edentulous or partially edentulous lower jaws received implant treatment. During second-stage surgery and prior to implant exposure, a vestibuloplasty was performed, using either FGG from the palate or a collagen matrix. The patients were followed up over a period of up to five years after surgery. Both groups revealed similar outcomes in terms of increase in KAM width, measuring 13.06 ± 2.26 mm in the FGG group and 12.96 ± 2.86 mm in the collagen matrix group. After six months, the width of keratinized mucosa had decreased to 67.08 ± 13.85% in the FGG group and 58.88 ± 14.62% in the collagen matrix group, with no statistically significant differences between the two groups. However, at five years, the total loss of the width of keratinized mucosa was statistically significant between the FGG (40.65%) and the collagen matrix group (52.89%), indicating higher long-term stability with the FGG. The findings suggested that both the FGG and a collagen matrix are suitable for gain of KAM at peri-implant sites, providing long-term stability.

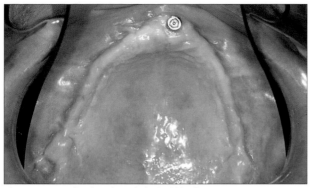

Fig 1   Preoperative situation. Limited width of KAM.

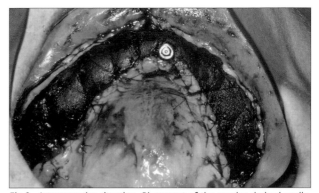

Fig 2   Intraoperative situation. Placement of the porcine-derived acellular dermal matrix (Mucoderm, Botiss, Berlin, Germany). The matrix was placed and sutured in direct contact with the remaining keratinized tissue on the palatal and buccal sides.

However, the collagen matrix yielded a more esthetic outcome than the FGG, with less surgical time and better patient acceptance.

In a recent prospective case series, Papi and Pompa (2018) evaluated the use of a porcine-derived acellular dermal matrix to improve the KAM around implants. Dental implants were placed in the upper premolar area in twelve patients. After eight weeks, a collagen matrix was placed during second-stage surgery. After one year, the mean KAM width was 5.67 ± 2.12 mm, thus indicating that the collagen matrix may represent a valuable modality to increase the width of the KAM at implants.

In a preclinical experimental model, Thoma and coworkers (2020) recently compared the efficacy of FGG, a collagen matrix, and an apically positioned flap alone for regenerating the KAM around implants. The results showed that the use of FGG demonstrated a higher tendency for KAM regeneration, although without statistically significant differences compared with the other treatments. Interestingly, the findings also suggested that the presence of a narrow band of keratinized tissue may have a positive influence on the final KAM gain.

These findings from animal studies are in line with the results of a clinical study evaluating the effectiveness and predictability of an apically positioned flap (APF) alone or combined with either a collagen matrix or FGG (Thoma and coworkers 2018b) in fully edentulous patients prior to implant placement. The results have shown that at three months after therapy, all three modalities resulted in a gain of KAM to a varying extent (1.93 ± 1.6 mm in the APF group, 4.63 ± 1.25 mm in the collagen matrix group, 3.64 ± 2.01 mm in the FGG group). The histologic analysis revealed a regular mucoperiosteal structure with a keratinized epithelium of comparable thickness in all groups. The results provided clinical and histological evidence that suggested that the use of xenogeneic soft-tissue replacement grafts in conjunction with an APF is a valuable treatment option to obtain a KAM at implants placed in edentulous sites.

Conclusion

The available evidence indicates that under certain circumstances (presence of a narrow band of KAM), soft-tissue replacement materials may represent a realistic option for KAM gain at implants (Figs 1 to 4 and Figs 5 to 8).

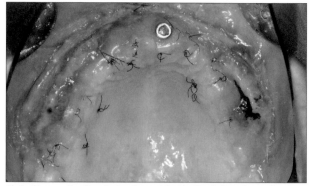

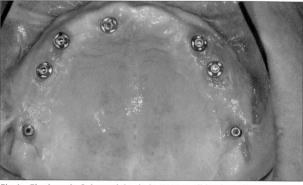

Fig 3   Two weeks after placing the matrix. Healing is free of complications. Incipient vascularization of the grafted area.

Fig 4   Final result. Substantial gain in KAM at all implant sites.

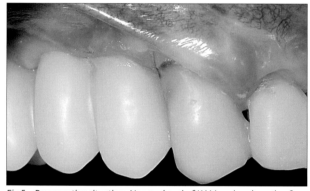

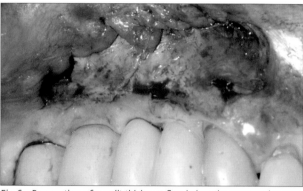

Fig 5   Preoperative situation. Narrow band of KAM and an inserting frenulum.

Fig 6   Preparation of a split-thickness flap below the preserved narrow band of KAM.

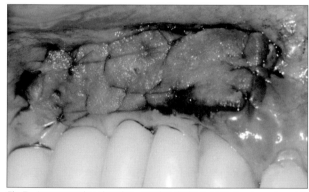

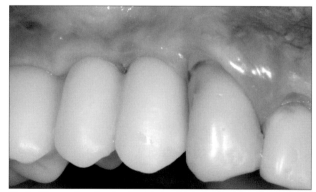

Fig 7   Intraoperative situation. Porcine-derived acellular dermal matrix sutured to the periosteum in direct contact with the remaining KAM.

Fig 8   Six months after treatment, a substantial gain in KAM is visible. The final prosthetic reconstruction will be placed later.

Figures 1 to 4 demonstrate the use of a porcine-derived acellular dermal matrix to increase KAM around implants (Fig 1). Following preparation of a split-thickness flap, a porcine derived acellular dermal matrix (Mucoderm, Botiss, Berlin, Germany) was attached to the periosteum and placed in contact with the palatal and vestibular keratinized tissue (Fig 2). The early healing at two weeks following placement of the matrix indicated complication-free clinical healing and ingrowth of blood vessels (Fig 3). The result indicates a substantial gain in KAM at all implant sites.

Acknowledgments

Surgical procedures, Figs. 1 to 4
Dr Bálint Molnár – Semmelweis University Budapest. Hungary

5 Peri-Implant Soft-Tissue Dehiscences

M. Roccuzzo, A. Sculean

5.1 Indications for Peri-Implant Soft-Tissue Dehiscence Coverage

M. Roccuzzo

A significant number of publications in the field of implant dentistry report high long-term implant survival rates (Adell and coworkers 1990; Lindquist and coworkers 1996; Wennström and coworkers 2005; Buser and coworkers 2012; Dierens and coworkers 2012; Chappuis and coworkers 2013; Quirynen and coworkers 2014; Roccuzzo and coworkers 2014a). Nevertheless, implant survival does not necessarily mean a successful esthetic and functional rehabilitation (Zucchelli and coworkers 2013b; Roccuzzo and coworkers 2014b). In the anterior maxilla and in other esthetic zones, the peri-implant soft tissues should be similar in appearance to the adjacent tissues at natural teeth in order to be esthetically acceptable. This may be more difficult to achieve with implant-supported restorations than with crowns on natural teeth. Moreover, while a soft-tissue recession around a tooth usually does not create an esthetic problem until it becomes significant, a soft-tissue recession around an implant can create an unacceptable appearance even if

it only amounts to 1 mm or less (Zucchelli and coworkers 2018a) (Fig 1).

An inconspicuous implant will always be accompanied by soft tissue in harmony with the adjacent natural teeth, including (Figs 2 and 3a-c):

- Intact interdental papillae
- A convex contour of the buccal soft tissue
- Scalloped mucosa
- Absence of mucosal pigmentation

The ideal appearance may be impaired by implant or abutment exposure, by a misalignment of the gingival margin, or by a "grayish" tint of the soft tissues where the underlying implant or abutment shows through the mucosa. In some circumstances, inappropriate hygiene techniques can also be a contributing factor, as in the case depicted in Figures 4a-e.

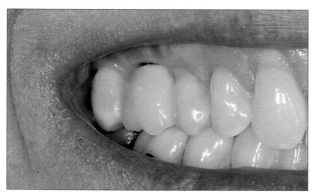

Fig 1   Even though a significant recession was present on the natural canine, with a recession associated with abrasion on the second premolar, the patient complained about the minimal soft-tissue dehiscence buccal to implant 16, which was visible when smiling.

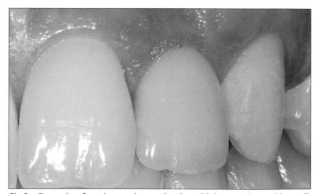

Fig 2   Example of an inconspicuous implant 22 in a patient with medium-thick tissue phenotype. The long-term risk of peri-implant soft-tissue dehiscence is limited.

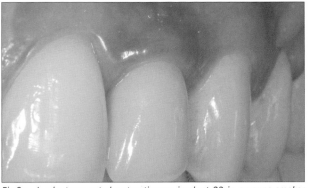

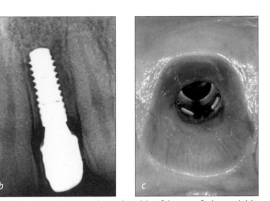

Fig 3a   Implant-supported restoration on implant 22 in a young smoker with thin tissue phenotype and gingival recession on the adjacent central incisor. The long-term risk of peri-implant soft-tissue dehiscence is elevated.

Fig 3b-c   In order to reduce the risk of later soft-tissue dehiscence, a reduced-diameter implant was selected. The surgical and prosthetic procedures were optimized to obtain a thick, firm, and healthy soft tissue around the collar of the implant, which was modeled before final impressions were taken.

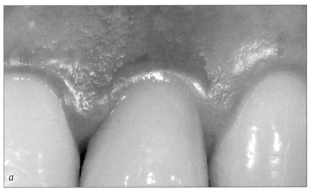

Figs 4a-b   Buccal view (a) and radiograph (b) at the time of delivery of the ceramic crown.

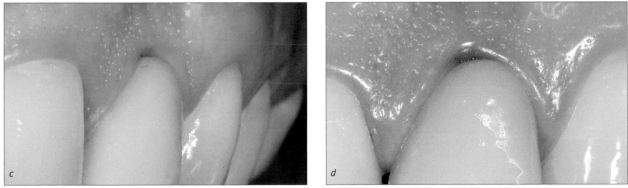

Figs 4c-d   Lateral and frontal view at five years. While the appearance of the mesial papilla has improved, a soft-tissue dehiscence has created a minor esthetic problem. Plaque control was not ideal. Surgical measures to achieve coverage were not considered at the time, but repeated instructions for proper and motivated oral hygiene were given.

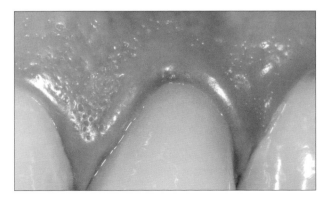

Fig 4e   Optimal peri-implant soft-tissue contours, at the fifteen-year follow-up. The patient regularly received supportive periodontal therapy; where needed, supragingival instrumentation was performed.

Table 1   Classification of peri-implant soft-tissue dehiscence/deficiencies (PSTD) and recommended surgical treatment (Zucchelli and coworkers 2019).

Class	Peri-implant soft-tissue dehiscence/deficiency characteristics	Recommended surgical treatment
I	The soft-tissue margin is located at the same level of the ideal position of the gingival margin of the homologous natural tooth, and the color of the abutment/implant is visible only through the mucosa and/or there is a lack of keratinized tissue/soft-tissue thickness	Ia: CAF or tunnel + CTG (or other graft substitutes) Ib: Combined prosthetic-surgical approach
II	The soft-tissue margin is located more apical to the ideal position of the gingival margin of the homologous natural tooth; and the implant-supported crown profile is located inside (more palatal) the imaginary curve line that connects the profile of the adjacent teeth at the level of the soft-tissue margin	IIa: No crown removal, CAF + CTG IIb: Combined prosthetic-surgical approach IIc: Soft-tissue augmentation with submerged healing
III	The soft-tissue margin is located more apical to the ideal position of the gingival margin of the homologous natural tooth The implant-supported crown profile is located outside (more facially) the imaginary curve line that connects the profile of the adjacent teeth at the level of the soft-tissue margin, and the head of the implant (evaluated by removing the crown) is inside (more palatally) the imaginary straight line connecting the profile of the adjacent teeth at the level of the soft-tissue margin	IIIa: Crown removal, CAF + CTG IIIb: Combined prosthetic-surgical approach. IIIc: Soft-tissue augmentation with submerged healing
IV	The soft-tissue margin is located more apical with respect of the ideal position of the gingival margin of the homologous natural tooth The implant-supported crown profile is located outside (more facially) the imaginary curve line that connects the profile of the adjacent teeth at the level of the soft-tissue margin, and the head of the implant (evaluated by removing the crown) is outside (more facially) the imaginary straight line connecting the profile of the adjacent teeth at the level of the soft-tissue margin	IVa: Combined prosthetic-surgical approach IVb: Soft-tissue augmentation with submerged healing IVc: Implant removal
Subclass		
a	The tip of both papillae is ≥ 3 mm coronal to the ideal position of soft-tissue margin of the implant-supported crown	
b	The tip of at least one papilla is ≥ 1 mm but < 3 mm coronal to the ideal position of the soft-tissue margin of the implant supported crown	
c*	The height of at least one papilla is < 1 mm coronal to the ideal position of the soft-tissue margin of the implant-supported crown	

*Does not apply to class I PSTD

Several differences between mucosal recessions occurring around teeth and implants should be highlighted.

For natural teeth, the definition of gingival recession is related to the presence of the cementoenamel junction (CEJ); a soft-tissue recession is defined as an apical shift of the margin away from the CEJ.

Around implants, there is no fixed reference point like the ones around natural teeth, so obtaining a standard measurement is more difficult. Hence, there is no agreed definition of peri-implant soft-tissue recession.

In 2018, the World Workshop on the Classification of Periodontal and Peri-Implant Diseases and Conditions endorsed a new classification of recessions around teeth (Cortellini and Bissada 2018). However, no consensus was reached on a classification of mucosal recession around implants, even though such a proposal was recently put forward by Zucchelli and coworkers (2019). According to them, since these complications can manifest themselves either as mucosal recession (apical shift of the peri-implant mucosal margin), as a grayish hue of the mucosa, or as discrepancies in the length of the implant-supported crown (compared with the homologous natural teeth), the term *peri-implant soft-tissue dehiscence/deficiency* (PSTD) may be the most appropriate (Table 1).

Four classes of PSTD are illustrated, based on the position of the gingival margin of the implant-supported crown in relation to the homologous natural tooth and the buccolingual position of the implant shoulder. Each class is further subdivided based on the height of the anatomical papillae.

One of the limitations of this classification is that it relies on the assumption that the homologous natural tooth is intact and in the proper anatomic position. A second limitation is that it includes only single peri-implant defects between adjacent teeth. As a result, a PSTD caused by an implant placed too far coronally, as in the case in Figures 5a-b, is not covered by this classification.

A third limitation of this classification is that even though it is meant to help clinicians select a particular surgical approach to revision, the "combined prosthetic-surgical approach" is recommended in all four classes, rendering decisions, on the basis of the classification only, difficult.

Before attempting to correct a peri-implant soft-tissue recession, the reasons and the time of occurrence of the problem must be assessed in a thorough analysis. Table 2 illustrates the main predisposing factors for the formation of soft-tissue dehiscences around implants.

Table 2 Predisposing factors for the formation of soft-tissue dehiscences around implants.

Facial osseous dehiscence/fenestration
Buccally positioned implant
Large-diameter implant/abutment
Thin gingival phenotype
Insufficient papilla height
Lack of keratinized tissue
High frenulum or muscle pull
Recurrent inflammation
Improperly performed oral hygiene
Smoking

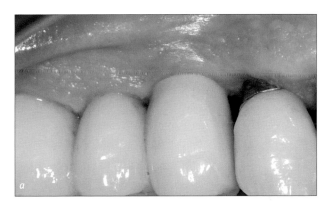

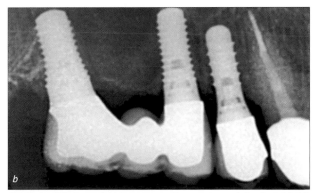

Figs 5a-b Soft-tissue dehiscence around a regular-neck implant 14 (a). The periapical radiograph shows that the implant was placed in a more coronal position, 2 mm above the level of the adjacent implant 15 (b).

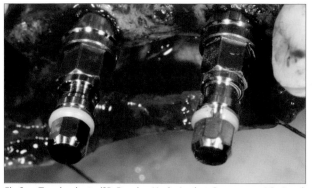

Fig 6a Two implants (SP Regular Neck, Institut Straumann AG, Basel, Switzerland) were placed at the sites of the first premolar and the first molar (teeth 14 and 16).

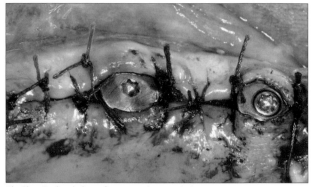

Fig 6b Occlusal view after non-submerged closure.

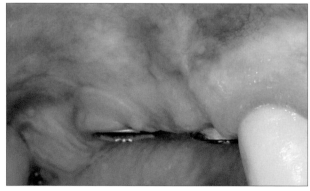

Fig 6c Lateral view at three months.

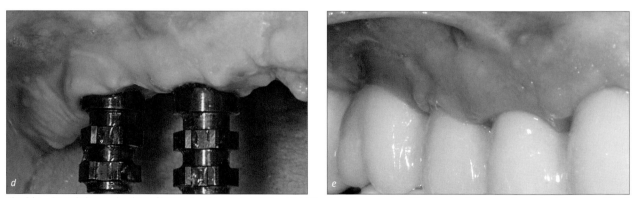

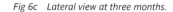

Figs 6d-e Buccal view at the time of impression (d) and at delivery (e) of the definitive ceramic bridge showing the mucosal margin at the correct level. The mucogingival line was not displaced.

Recessions around implants can be found with both correctly placed implants (Fig 6) and around implants placed in an inappropriate position, whether due to poor planning or due to a lack of surgical experience. Implant placement in a reduced horizontal bone dimension may increase the risk of mucosal recession, even in the presence of an intact but thin buccal cortical bone plate. In fact, bone remodeling following surgical procedures may result in vertical buccal bone loss with exposure of the coronal portion of the implant, which may cause a mucosal recession in the long term. Just as with natural teeth, a thin tissue phenotype constitutes an additional risk of for mucosal recession (Evans and Chen 2008). Figures 6a-m show a case, originally published in the ITI Treatment Guide, Volume 7, of a soft-tissue recession facially to a properly positioned implant.

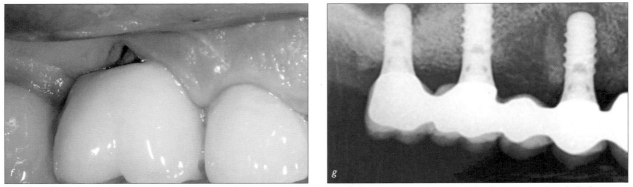

Figs 6f-g   Clinical and radiographic situation six years after implant placement. A soft-tissue dehiscence is visible at implant 16 even though the interprox-imal bone level is normal.

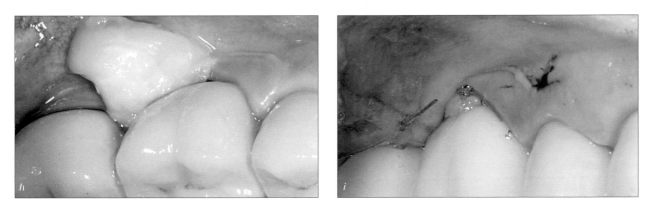

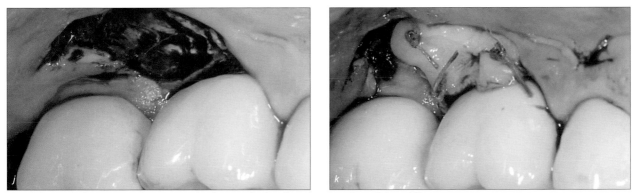

Figs 6h-k   Surgical treatment using a connective-tissue graft taken from the tuberosity and shaped like a pentagon.

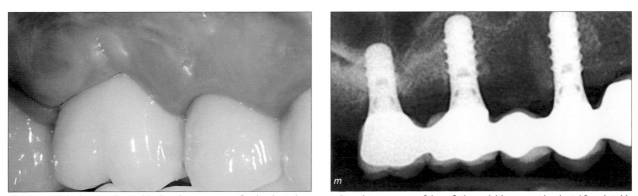

Fig 6l-m   Clinical and radiographic situation ten years after implant placement. Complete coverage of the soft-tissue dehiscence at implant 16 and stable interproximal bone levels.

Peri-implant soft-tissue dehiscences are more frequently found around implants placed in an incorrect three-dimensional position or at an inappropriate angle. The incidence of such errors is typically higher in the anterior maxilla with implants immediately placed into extraction sockets (Chen and Buser 2014). Figures 7a-d illustrate one such case, which was subsequently successfully resolved.

For this reason, it was suggested during the 3rd ITI Consensus Conference that when treating patients with a thin, scalloped gingival phenotype—even those with an intact buccal plate—concomitant augmentation at the time of placement (type 1) is recommended because of the high risk of buccal-plate resorption and marginal tissue recession (Hämmerle and coworkers 2004).

Chen and coworkers (2007) were among the first to demonstrate the risk of mucosal recession and adverse soft-tissue esthetics with immediate implant placement. Buccal mucosal recession was observed to be significantly associated with a more buccal implant position in a prospective cohort study of 30 implants. These findings were confirmed in a retrospective study with 42 single implants in the esthetic zone, reporting a significant association of buccal mucosal recession with buccal implant positioning (Evans and Chen 2008). Another retrospective study photographically analyzed the level of the mucosal margin at 85 single-tooth implants, after immediate placement without flap elevation in the esthetic zone, compared to the reference central incisor (Chen and coworkers 2009). The procedure was found to be associated with recession of the marginal mucosa. Furthermore, the orofacial position of the implant shoulder and the tissue phenotype were considered important contributory factors.

Cosyn and coworkers (2012) presented a systematic review on the frequency of advanced recession following immediate single implant placement. The authors concluded that soft-tissue recession may be expected following implant placement in extraction sockets; multiple factors seemed to contribute to the phenomenon. Furthermore, they encouraged a proper generic risk assessment addressing diagnostic, surgical, and restorative aspects to avoid compromised outcomes.

The consensus report and clinical recommendations of Group 3 of the XV European Workshop in Periodontology 2019 (Tonetti and coworkers 2019) regarding the management of the extraction socket and timing of implant placement were based on a systematic review by Cosyn and coworkers (2019). In this review, no significant conclusions were delivered because the vast majority of the included studies underreported the soft-tissue recession, and the available data were highly biased. The group was only able to conclude that the presence of a thin periodontal phenotype or a high smile line in subjects with high esthetic expectations represents an unfavorable scenario for immediate or early implant placement in extraction sockets. In such situations, alveolar-ridge preservation via socket grafting and delayed or late implant placement should be considered to reduce the risk of peri-implant soft-tissue dehiscence.

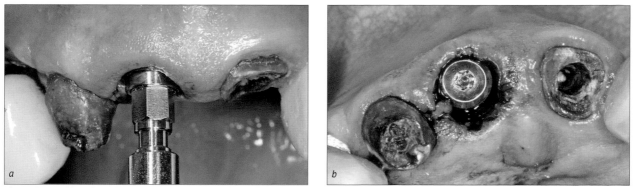

Figs 7a-b   Implant placed immediately into an extraction socket with excessive buccal inclination.

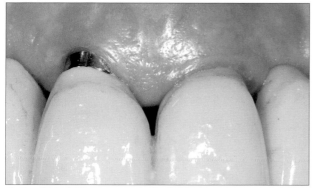

Fig 7c   Clinical view one year after implant placement.

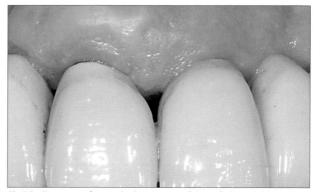

Fig 7d   Ten years after surgical treatment of the soft-tissue dehiscence.

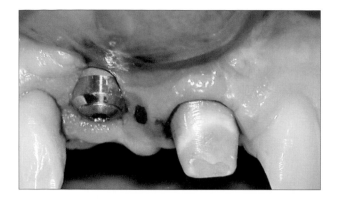

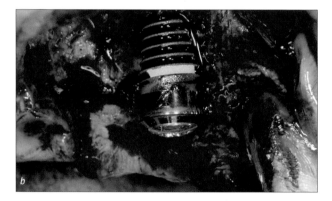

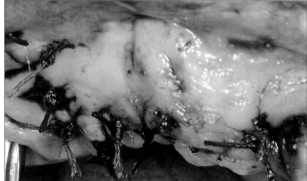

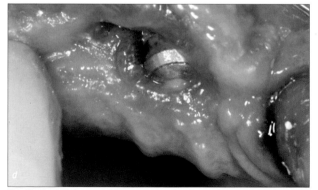

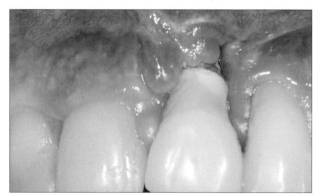

Fig 8a   Soft-tissue dehiscence as a consequence of mesiodistal and orofacial malpositioning, a few weeks after surgery. The implant is too close to the lateral incisor, with a subsequently reduction in papilla height, and too far towards the facial aspect, with insufficient buccal bone supporting the soft tissues, with hard- and soft-tissue recession as a consequence.

Figs 8b-d   Soft-tissue dehiscence after implant placement and guided bone regeneration. The most common reason for this type of complication is related to a not completely tension-free flap closure.

Fig 8e   Patient referred for coverage of a soft-tissue dehiscence. Two failed attempts at soft-tissue grafting had already been made subsequent to implant placement. Considering the amount of soft-tissue destruction, explantation was suggested.

Peri-implant recession can appear shortly after surgery (Fig 8a-e) and are then usually considered as a surgical complication. Typically, such situations are not predictably corrected by surgery; in most cases, implant removal may be required. In these circumstances, it is important to avoid a perceived need for prompt intervention, as this often initiates a cycle of multiple ineffective surgical attempts.

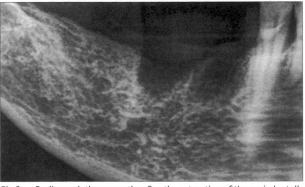

Fig 9a   Radiograph three months after the extraction of the periodontally compromised premolars.

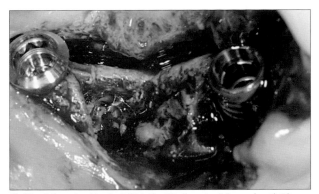

Fig 9b   A tissue-level implant (SLActive SP, diameter 3.3 mm, length 10 mm; Institut Straumann AG) was placed at site 46, while a bone-level implant (SLActive BL RC, diameter 4.1 mm, length 12 mm; Institut Straumann AG) was preferred for site 44, in conjunction with vertical bone regeneration.

At other times, a soft-tissue recession may appear during healing, before definitive prosthetic loading—even around properly placed implants. This may occur when the clinician does not take into consideration the inevitable shrinkage of the soft tissues, particularly after suboptimal bone regeneration (Fontana and coworkers 2011). Depending on the circumstances, successful treatment of such soft-tissue defects may not be possible. The predictability of successfully covering recession defects depends on several factors, in particular on the size of the dehiscence and the amount of hard- and soft-tissue loss. Figures 9a-m illustrate a successful treatment of such a defect, of limited size.

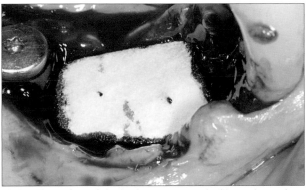

Fig 9c   The surface of the implant was covered with autologous bone chips and DBBM particles, protected by a native collagen membrane of porcine origin (Collprotect; Botiss Biomaterials, Zossen, Germany)

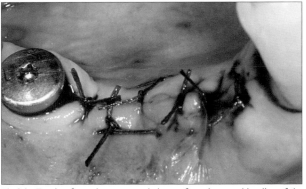

Fig 9d   Tension-free primary wound closure for submerged healing of the more mesial implant. The flap was sutured with a horizonal mattress suture and multiple interrupted sutures.

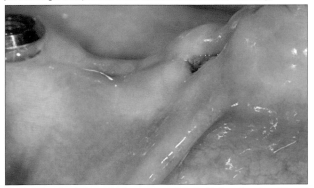

Fig 9e   Small soft-tissue dehiscence associated with frenulum insertion, at four weeks.

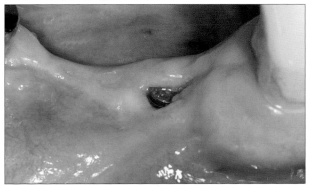

Fig 9f   At the two-month follow-up, the dehiscence had grown, suggesting the need for soft-tissue augmentation before the delivery of the final restoration.

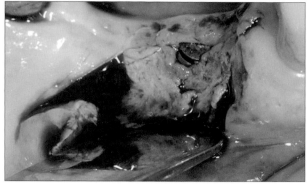

Fig 9g   The surgical procedure was initiated with a trapezoidal split-thickness flap.

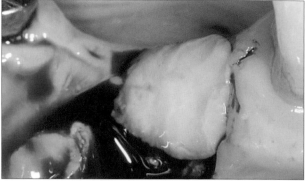

Fig 9h   The head of the implant was covered with a wide connective-tissue graft.

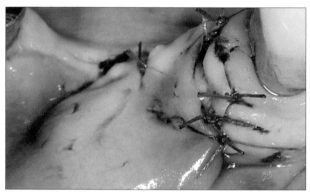

Fig 9i   The flap was coronally displaced and sutured (4-0 Vicryl) for complete coverage of the implant.

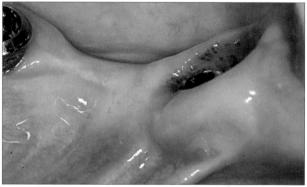

Fig 9j   Optimal healing of the peri-implant soft tissue at the time of impression-taking for definitive prosthesis.

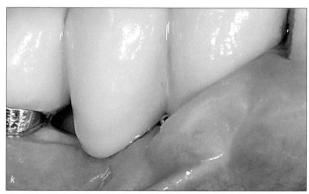

Figs 9k-l   Clinical (k) and radiographic (l) images of the three-unit screw-retained metal-ceramic bridge.

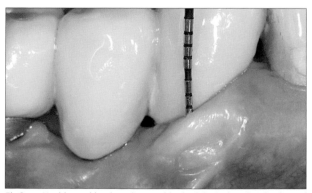

Fig 9m   Healthy peri-implant tissues with physiological pocket depths and no bleeding on probing at the three-year follow-up.

In some situations, soft-tissue marginal recession with consequent exposure of the titanium may arise several years after implant placement. This may be because, with time, there will be some resorption of a thin buccal bone crest, which produces—especially in patients with a thin tissue phenotype—an apical shift of the soft-tissue cuff. Apart from the esthetic problems this may cause, the treatment of peri-implant recessions may be indicated from a subsequent exposure to the oral environment of the rough portion of the implant (Figs 10a-b).

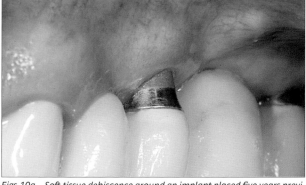

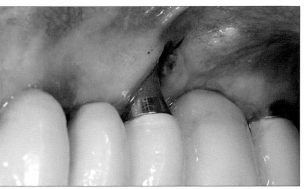

Figs 10a   Soft-tissue dehiscence around an implant placed five years previously. Since it was not an esthetic issue for the patient, the patient declined the proposed surgery for the coverage of the rough portion of the implant.

Fig 10b   Two years later. Increase in the size of the soft-tissue recession, with inflammation.

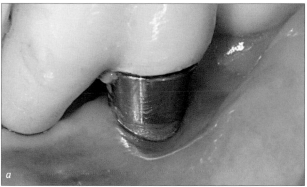

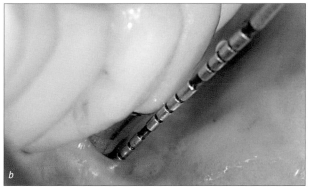

Figs 11a-b   Ten years after implant placement. Plaque control is not ideal due to insufficient vestibular depth and the absence of keratinized tissue. Exposed rough surface of the implant and mobility of the mucosal margin.

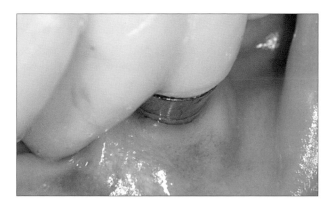

Fig 11c   Three years after treatment of the soft-tissue dehiscence with a connective-tissue graft. Complete coverage of the rough surface of the implant was achieved; the patient's own plaque control had improved.

Most implants today have a microrough surface, produced with various techniques such as sandblasting or acid etching to provide significantly enhanced initial bone-to-implant contact (BIC) and a higher removal torque during the early healing period compared to older machined implant surfaces (Li and coworkers 2002; Ferguson and coworkers 2006). The benefits include shorter healing times and a lower percentage of early failures in soft bone (type IV).

However, these surfaces may be more easily colonized by bacteria present in the oral cavity, particularly if the mucosal margin is mobile and there is no effective soft-tissue seal around the implant (Louropoulou and coworkers 2012). In a recent in-vitro study, Bermejo and coworkers (2019) found that implants with moderately rough surfaces accumulated more bacterial biomass and significant higher numbers of pathogenic bacteria (such as F. nucleatum and A. actinomycetemcomitans) than implants with smooth surfaces in a similar biofilm environment. It may thus seem reasonable to attempt soft-tissue coverage of the rough portion of the implant to reduce the risk of biological complications, even in cases where there is no esthetic concern (Figs 11a-c).

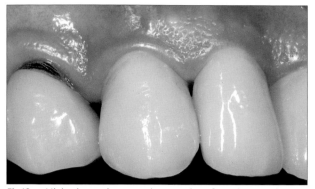

Fig 12a   Minimal recession around a smooth surface abutment in a patient with very low esthetic expectations (December 2007).

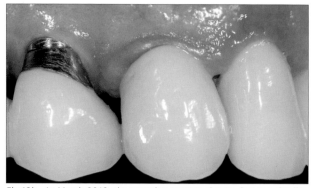

Fig 12b   In March 2019, the recession appears deeper, but remains limited to the smooth coronal portion of the implant. The patient is unconcerned and declined treatment.

If, however, the portion of the implant/abutment exposed to the oral cavity is smooth, any necessity for treatment is almost entirely esthetic in nature. Esthetic perception varies a great deal from patient to patient (Figs 12a-b).

Every time a clinician encounters a soft-tissue recession, it is important to assess whether it may be associated with a biological complication, either peri-implant mucositis (Heitz-Mayfield and Salvi 2018a) or peri-implantitis (Schwarz and coworkers 2018).

According to the 2017 World Workshop on the Classification of Periodontal and Peri-implant Diseases and Conditions, peri-implant mucositis is characterized by bleeding on probing and visual signs of inflammation. While there is strong evidence that peri-implant mucositis is caused by plaque, there is very limited evidence for non-plaque-induced peri-implant mucositis. Peri-implant mucositis can be reversed with measures aimed at eliminating the plaque. Peri-implantitis was defined as a plaque-associated pathologic condition occurring in the tissue around implants, characterized by inflammation in the peri-implant mucosa and a subsequent progressive loss of supporting bone. Peri-implant mucositis is assumed to precede peri-implantitis. Peri-implantitis is associated with poor plaque control and with patients with a history of severe periodontitis (Caton and coworkers 2018).

Once etiological factors are eliminated and adequate plaque control is performed, it is possible to attempt restoration of the initial peri-implant tissue situation. Clinicians must, however, be aware that the initial treatment of biological complications may lead to increased soft-tissue dehiscence as in the clinical case presented in Figures 13a-b.

When a peri-implant soft-tissue dehiscence is associated with severe bone loss, particularly in multiple adjacent sites, treatment is not predictable and implant removal may be the only available option (Figs 14a-b).

The successful surgical treatment of peri-implantitis often produces recession of the soft-tissue margin, affecting esthetics, phonetics, and comfort during oral hygiene (Roccuzzo and coworkers 2017b). Complications of this kind have been documented in two recent studies (Heitz-Mayfield and coworkers 2018b; Mercado and coworkers 2018). Such factors are highly relevant to clinical decision-making and should be discussed with patients before initiating treatment.

In some instances, peri-implant mucositis will already be present. Here, the rationale for additional soft-tissue treatment is based on the possibility of obtaining better anatomical conditions for subsequent optimal plaque control. The decision on whether to remove the implant

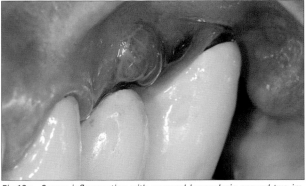

Fig 13a Severe inflammation with mucosal hyperplasia around two implants in the maxilla.

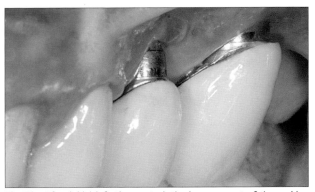

Fig 13b After initial infection control, the improvement of the peri-implant soft tissue was accompanied by significant shrinkage, with exposure of the abutments and portions of the titanium implants.

or attempt to treat the complication is often a difficult one, as it cannot be based on validated guidelines or consensus statements. Consequently, the decision should rely on a good understanding of the biological mechanisms of wound healing, combined with a thorough discussion of any treatment alternatives with the patient. The coverage of peri implant recessions is a relatively new topic, and most published studies are case series with a limited number of subjects. As the possibility of achieving an optimal esthetic result may be challenging, the clinician should take into consideration, together with all relevant evaluations, the patient's expectations, particularly in patients with high esthetic demands, and review all available treatment alternatives.

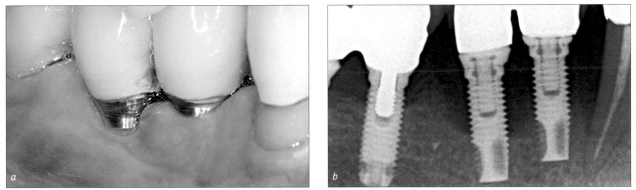

Figs 14a-b Clinical (a) and radiographic (b) images of two implants with mucosal recession associated with severe bone loss due to peri-implantitis and periodontitis, indicating unsuitability for treatment of the soft-tissue dehiscence.

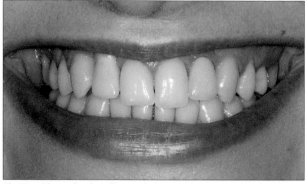

Fig 15a   The patient's smile revealed a grayish area apical to implant 22 and a poor pink-ceramic restoration in the cervical area of crown 12.

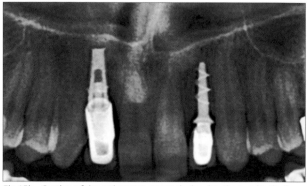

Fig 15b   Section of the orthopantomograph showing the two implants.

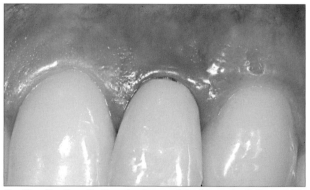

Figs 15c   Baseline situation showing a minimal buccal soft-tissue dehiscence affecting the implant-supported crown 22; the abutment shines through the soft tissue.

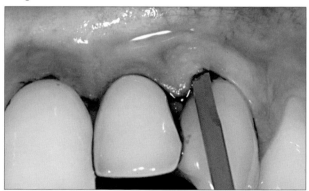

Fig 15d   A single horizontal incision was performed with a micro blade, with no vertical releasing incisions.

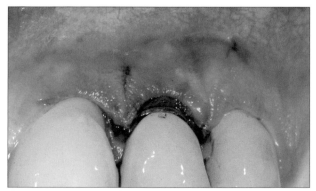

Fig 15e   A split-thickness flap was elevated and the anatomic papillae de-epithelialized.

Figures 15a-m and 16a-j illustrate the case of a 25-year-old woman previously treated with implants at sites 12 and 22, who was referred by her lawyer during litigation with her previous dentist over the poor esthetic outcome.

The patient's chief complaint was the unesthetic appearance of the two implant-supported crowns (Fig 15a). Implant 22 had been placed more than a year before and presented with no clinical or radiological signs of peri-implant mucositis or peri-implantitis (Fig 15b). The soft-tissue margin of the implant-supported crown was located more apical than the ideal position of the gingival margin when compared to the corresponding natural tooth (Fig 15c). The possible treatment alternatives were thoroughly discussed with the patient.

A decision was made to keep implant 22 and to treat the problem. A split-thickness flap was elevated via a single horizontal incision with no vertical releasing incisions. The anatomic papillae were de-epithelialized. A gingival cuff was excised by a gingivectomy from the tuberosity area. It was de-epithelialized with a blade and trimmed with a mucotome to obtain a U-shape to facilitate optimal adaptation to the implant collar (Roccuzzo and coworkers 2014b). The graft was approximately 3 mm thick. It was inserted into the pouch and secured at the base of the anatomical papillae with two resorbable interrupted sutures. The flap was gently mobilized until the soft-tissue margin reached a level coronal to the connective-tissue graft and then sutured (5-0 Vicryl) in a coronal position to cover the graft with minimal tension. The sutures were kept in place for two weeks. The patient was instructed not to disturb the treated area and to rinse for 1 minute with a 0.12% chlorhexidine solution three times a day for three weeks.

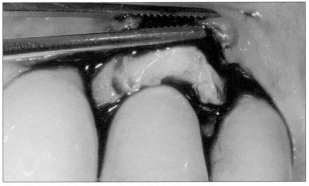

Fig 15f   The thick graft was inserted into the pouch.

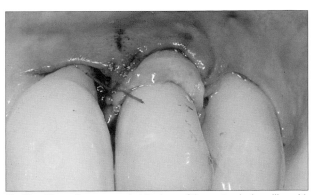

Fig 15g   The graft was secured at the base of the anatomical papillae with two resorbable interrupted sutures.

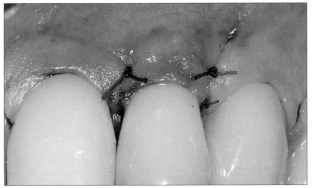

Fig 15h   The flap was mobilized and sutured with 5-0 Vicryl in a coronal position to cover the graft with minimal tension.

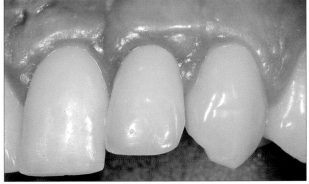

Fig 15i   At fifteen months.

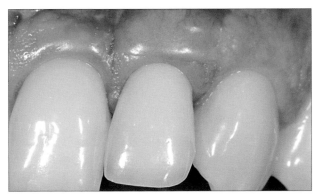

Fig 15j   At three years.

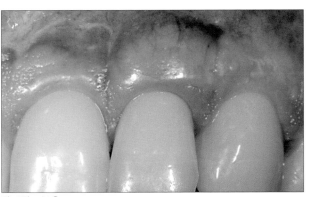

Fig 15k   At five years.

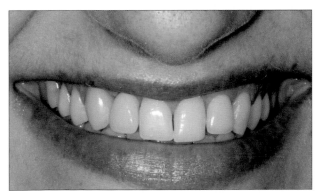

Fig 15l   The patient's smile after surgical treatment.

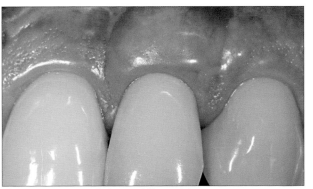

Fig 15m   Long-term soft-tissue stability at eight years.

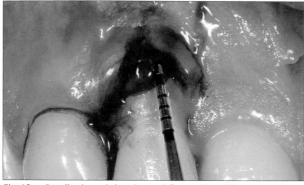

Figs 16a   Baseline buccal view. Severe inflammation with edema and profuse bleeding on probing around implant 12.

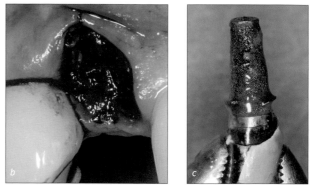

Figs 16b-c   The implant was removed. Due to the significant infection on the site, grafting was postponed until later.

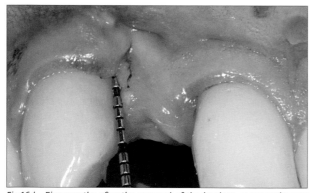

Fig 16d   Five months after the removal of the implant, a concavity was evident at site 12, with significant periodontal attachment loss mesial to the canine.

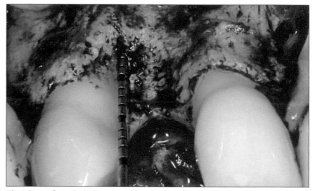

Fig 16e   After elevating a mucoperiosteal flap, a large vertical and horizontal bone defect was visible.

On the right side, since the esthetic problem was associated with peri-implantitis, it was decided to remove the implant, accepting that further bone loss would inevitably follow (Fig 16a). Since the implant could not be replaced immediately, consideration was given to reconstructing the site to allow a replacement later (Fig 16b), even though the literature on bone augmentation after implant removal is limited. It was decided to wait several months to assure optimal soft-tissue maturation (Fig 16c).

Site reconstruction followed the established principles of GBR, starting with the elevation of a large trapezoidal full-thickness flap (Fig 16d). Analysis of the site revealed the loss of periodontal support on both adjacent teeth. To promote periodontal regeneration, Emdogain (Institut Straumann AG) was applied on the roots of 11 and 13 (Fig 16e). An autologous bone block was harvested from the external oblique ridge and split into two parts. One part was secured in place with three screws. The other

half was milled to create bone chips to facilitate void-free adaptation between the block and the recipient site (Fig 16f). To minimize postsurgical graft resorption, the block was covered with deproteinized bovine bone mineral (Bio-Oss; Geistlich, Wolhusen, Switzerland), protected by a collagen membrane (Bio-Gide; Geistlich), and left to heal for five months (Figs 16g-j).

After an undisturbed healing period, an excellent bone regeneration outcome allowed optimal positioning of a bone level implant (BL NC SLActive Roxolid, diameter 3.3 mm, length 10 mm; Institut Straumann AG). To minimize postsurgical soft-tissue shrinkage, a connective-tissue graft was placed on the facial aspect of the canine for contour augmentation and papilla support (Figs 16k-m). After several months of soft-tissue maturation with a provisional restoration, a ceramic crown was delivered (Figs 16n-r).

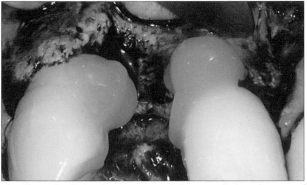

Fig 16f   Emdogain (Institut Straumann AG) was applied on the roots of teeth 11 and 13 to promote periodontal regeneration.

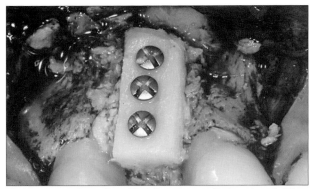

Fig 16g   An autologous bone block from the mandibular external oblique ridge was harvested and stabilized using three screws. The voids between the recipient site and the block were filled with bone chips.

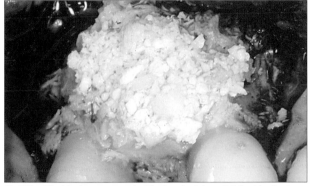

Fig 16h   The block was covered with abundant deproteinized bovine bone mineral in order to reduce graft resorption.

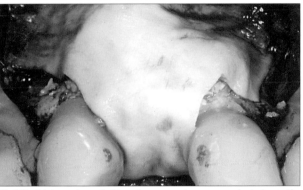

Fig 16i   A trimmed resorbable collagen membrane was adapted over the grafted area.

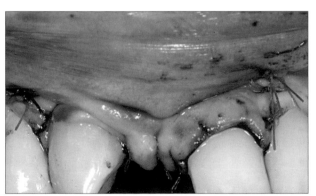

Fig 16j   Coronally advanced flap for tension-free primary wound closure.

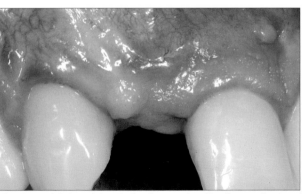

Fig 16k   Facial view of site 12 after five months of healing, on the day of implant surgery.

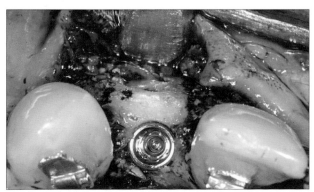

Fig 16l   Occlusal view of site 12 following the insertion of the implant.

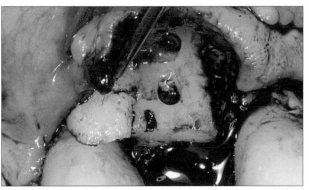

Fig 16m   A connective-tissue graft was placed on the facial aspect of the canine for contour augmentation and papilla support.

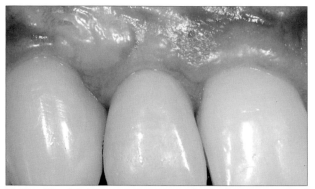

Fig 16n   The definitive crown, one year after implant surgery. Good soft-tissue volume and papilla height.

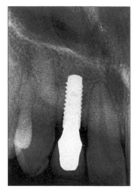

Fig 16o   Periapical radiograph. The implant two years after surgery.

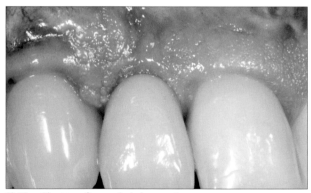

Fig16p   Six years after surgical placement.

If a soft-tissue dehiscence has caused an esthetic complication, the dentist faces the dilemma of having to decide if surgical therapy to maintain the implant should be attempted or removal and replacement with a new implant would be preferred. While no clear guidelines exist for deciding when an implant with a soft-tissue dehiscence should be removed, the ITI Treatment Guide Volume 10 (Chappuis and Martin 2017b) suggested the following factors be considered:

- Esthetic failure
- Implant mobility
- Peri-implantitis
- Implant fracture
- Implant malposition
- Pain
- Local pathology
- Psychological problems
- Damage to the prosthetic interface
- Obsolete components/implants

If mobility, fracture or peri-implantitis are present, it is imperative to remove the implant swiftly, before significant bone loss can occur that may jeopardize the chances for placing a new implant or may damage adjacent teeth, as in the clinical case illustrated in Figures 16a-r.

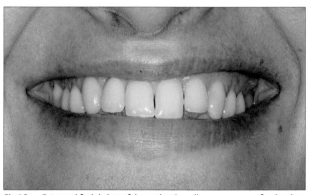

Fig 16q   Extraoral facial view of the patient's smile, seven years after implant placement, demonstrating a pleasing esthetic result for both treated sites.

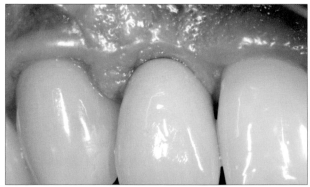

Fig 16r   Long-term soft-tissue stability, including the distal papilla, at eight years.

If the soft-tissue defect is associated with one of the other conditions, soft-tissue grafting may be attempted using one of the techniques proposed in the literature and presented in Chapter 5.2. The variability in the obtainable outcomes does not only depend on the surgical approach, but also on the case selection. Thus, it is critical to differentiate between the types of soft-tissue dehiscences before surgery, even though a comprehensive validated classification of the defects is not available at this stage.

Table 3 enumerates some parameters to be considered when evaluating the possibility of treating a soft-tissue dehiscence versus implant removal, with some clinical examples.

Finally, the decision between performing a surgical procedure to correct a soft-tissue defect or removing the implant must be rigorously based on patient's expectations and the surgeon's skills, having in mind that the correction of peri-implant soft-tissue deficiencies constitutes a major clinical challenge, particularly at sites that present deep defects and abundant interproximal tissue loss (Fig 17).

Table 3   Parameters of consideration for soft-tissue dehiscence treatment around dental implants.

Implant position	Interproximal tissue	Suggested treatment
Center of the crest	Present	Connective-tissue graft
Slightly buccal	Present or partly missing	Connective-tissue graft and new restoration
Center of the crest	Absent	Implant removal
Fully buccal	—	Implant removal

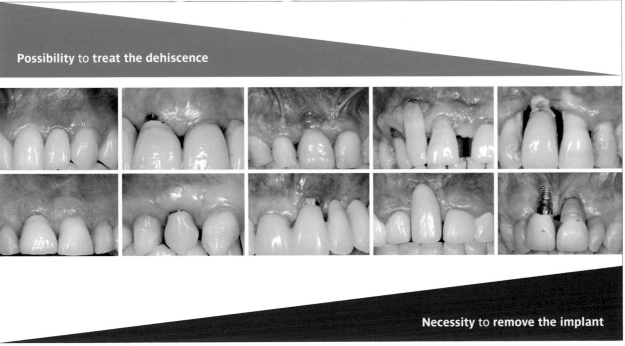

Possibility to **treat the dehiscence**

Necessity to **remove the implant**

Fig 17   Visual consultation matrix.

5.2 Techniques for Treating Peri-Implant Soft-Tissue Dehiscences

M. Roccuzzo

Treatment modalities

Several surgical and restorative techniques have been recently proposed for the treatment of peri-implant soft-tissue dehiscences. However, there is no evidence to suggest which of these treatment approaches is the most effective and predictable. The main reason for this is that neither Consensus Conferences nor systematic reviews on mucogingival therapy have been devoted to the presentation of the best available treatment of peri-implant dehiscences, due to the paucity of articles on the topic. A comprehensive research of the relevant literature has yielded descriptions of a variety of procedures, but most are case reports and only a few are prospective studies. It is not possible to draw any definitive conclusions from the literature, as each paper presents defects associated with different clinical situations (Sculean and coworkers 2017; Mazzotti and coworkers 2018).

The techniques most commonly described in the literature use connective-tissue grafts (CTG) with coronally advanced flaps. A major difference between the various studies is that some authors describe only surgical techniques, while others present a combination of surgical and restorative methods, including crown removal and, in some cases, abutment removal.

One of the critical aspects of an esthetically successful outcome of any implant treatment is the correct restoration-driven 3D implant position, replacing the tooth in a natural position and emulating a natural emergence profile (Belser and coworkers 2004; Buser and coworkers 2004).

Another critical aspect is the selection of the abutment. Implant treatment in the esthetic zone requires a careful choice of abutment, based on several factors such as the position of the adjacent and opposing teeth, the tissue phenotype, and the smile line. When a peri-implant soft-tissue dehiscence develops in a patient with high esthetic demands, the clinician has to decide whether to remove the prosthetic component, taking into account the cost and duration of the available treatment options.

In the absence of precise guidelines, the patient's viewpoint must also be considered. Complete coverage of a soft-tissue dehiscence will, in most circumstances, be the only acceptable outcome.

Combined surgical and restorative treatment

The first case report on the treatment of a peri-implant soft-tissue dehiscence was published by Mathews (2002), who described the treatment of unesthetic implant-supported restorations using a pedunculated CTG. Congenitally missing lateral incisors had been replaced with two apically and buccally malpositioned implants. The crowns were removed and small cover screws placed; these were substituted after two months with 2-mm healing abutments. A pedunculated CTG was performed on both sites, suturing them into labial split-thickness pouches about 3 mm apically to the implant platforms. Grafts were harvested from the regions of the first molars. The width of each graft was determined by the size of the site to be augmented and by the palatal vault depth. Four months after surgery, the healing abutments were uncovered by means of tissue punches. Three months later, screw-retained provisional crowns were positioned and left in place for three months. Finally, definitive ceramic crowns were placed. The author suggested that the pedunculated CTG was an excellent technique for vertical and labial augmentation of soft tissue to improve peri-implant esthetics.

Two years later, Shibli and coworkers (2004) described the use of a subepithelial CTG to recontour a soft-tissue margin discrepancy near an implant-supported single crown in the anterior maxilla. Before the surgical procedure, a new angled abutment was selected to minimize the influence of the abutment margin on soft-tissue healing after the surgery. A combined full- and partial-thickness trapezoidal flap was elevated with two vertical incisions and the epithelial tissue at the mesial and distal papillae was removed. The donor graft was obtained from the palate. The epithelial layer was removed; only the connective tissue was used. The graft was placed onto the polished abutment surface and stabilized with resorbable sutures. The flap was then coronally repositioned, fully covering the graft, and secured with interrupted sutures to avoid excessive tension. An interim prosthesis was fabricated and delivered with minimal contact with the peri-implant soft-tissue margin.

Six weeks after surgery, an implant-level impression was taken and the resulting definitive cast used for abutment selection and crown design. A second interim prosthesis was prepared on the definitive cast to develop a new emergence profile for the definitive restoration. This interim prosthesis was highly polished so as not to jeopardize the health of the peri-implant soft tissue. The second interim prosthesis was left in place until the definitive restoration was complete. Twelve weeks after the surgery, the definitive impression was taken using an individual resin coping. As the long axis of the implant had a slight buccal inclination, a prosthetic design with a cemented crown on a modified abutment was selected. The final shape of the abutment was designed to agree with the long axis of the implant and guided by the surfaces of the adjacent teeth. The abutment shoulder was prepared approximately 2 mm below the gingival level, following the contour of the gingival margin. A definitive metal-ceramic restoration was finally fabricated. The procedure was successful and provided an esthetic improvement with stable peri-implant soft tissues over a follow-up period of eighteen months.

Another two years later, Shibli and d'Avila (2006) reported the correction of an esthetic problem in two implant-supported single crowns using a subepithelial CTG while re-establishing a new abutment margin and crown emergence profile. Both cases presented an acceptable position and contour of both papillae, while the soft-tissue margin labial to the implant restoration was located further apically than the gingival margin on the adjacent natural tooth. Prior to surgery, a new abutment was selected to minimize the influence of the abutment margin on soft-tissue healing after the surgery, and an interim

prosthesis was placed to provide for a new soft-tissue profile during the healing period. A subepithelial CTG was placed onto the polished abutment surface and the prepared recipient tissue bed and stabilized with two interproximal and one apical resorbable 4-0 suture. The flap was coronally repositioned to fully cover the graft and secured with interrupted sutures to avoid excessive tension. Three months after the surgery, an impression was taken, and a second interim prosthesis was prepared on the master cast to develop a new emergence profile for the final restoration. Five months after the surgery, the final impression was taken and a metal-ceramic restoration fabricated. At the two-year follow-up, the adjacent peri-implant soft tissues were stable, and the peri-implant mucosal margin was located 2 to 3 mm further coronally, at the same level as on the adjacent central incisor.

Lai and coworkers (2010) first described the resubmergence technique to manage a soft-tissue dehiscence at an implant site 21 that developed a mucosal recession after being used for orthodontic anchorage. Marginal mucosal recession with exposure of the metal collar on the labial surface of the implant and 1 mm of further gingival recession at the labial surface of tooth 22 were noted. The author decided to remove the crown and abutment, later followed by elevating a partial-thickness flap. A cover screw was reattached to the implant and a subepithelial CTG harvested and sutured to cover the shoulder and buccal surface of the implant. The flap was coronally repositioned and closed with interrupted sutures. A provisional removable prosthesis was supplied for use during the recovery period. The implant was uncovered after two months using a tissue punch technique. The abutment with the provisional crown was reattached. The definitive metal-ceramic crown was delivered six months later.

Happe and coworkers (2013) presented a surgical approach to peri-implant soft-tissue discoloration caused by the shine-through effects of restorative materials at one single implant-supported crown, in the anterior maxilla. A minimally invasive tunneling approach and a CTG were used. A vertical access incision was created approximately 3 mm apical to the soft-tissue margin at the distal line angle of the implant-supported crown. The labial soft tissue was undermined using a split-thickness approach, resulting in a pouch that extended to the soft-tissue margin coronally and over the mucogingival junction apically. The CTG was inserted into the pouch and the access incision was secured by suturing. The spectrophotometric follow-up revealed an objective esthetic improvement at one year.

The first prospective pilot study was published by Zucchelli and coworkers (2013a). It included 20 patients with buccal soft-tissue dehiscences around single implants in the esthetic zone using a prosthetic/surgical/prosthetic approach. The preliminary negative results reported by Burkhardt and coworkers (2008) encouraged researchers to look for alternative approaches to overcome the limitations of the traditional approach, standard mucogingival surgery around teeth. The rationale was to increase the recipient area mesial and distal to the implant and to minimize the size of the abutment. Zucchelli and coworkers were the first to use the length of the clinical crown of the contralateral tooth as a benchmark to define treatment success.

Figures 1a-l show the technique as exemplified by a 32-year-old male patient whose chief complaint was the unesthetic length of the implant-supported crown when smiling. The implant had been placed eighteen months previously; no clinical or radiological signs of mucositis/peri-implantitis were detected. The soft-tissue margin of the implant-supported crown was located further apically than the ideal position of the gingival margin on the homologous natural tooth (Fig 1a). The tip of the distal papilla was up to 3 mm coronal to the ideal position of the soft-tissue margin. The crown profile was located inside the imaginary curve connecting the profile of the adjacent teeth (i.e., further palatally), at the level of the soft-tissue margin (Fig 1b). According to the new classification proposed by Zucchelli and coworkers (2019) the case was defined as a class 2, subclass b.

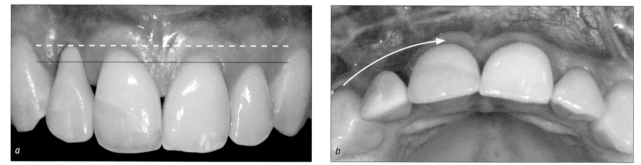

Figs 1a-b Baseline buccal and occlusal situation eighteen months after implant placement. Buccal soft-tissue dehiscence affecting the implant-supported crown 12.

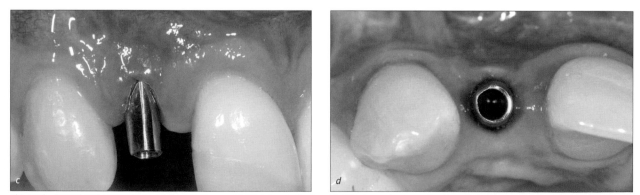

Figs 1c-d Buccal and occlusal view of the soft tissues after the pre-surgical prosthetic phase. A pre-surgical prosthetic phase comprised the removal of the implant-supported crown, reduction of the underlying abutment, and placement of a short provisional crown to improve the weak papillae. The increase in interdental soft tissue that could be de-epithelialized toward the palatal aspect helped ensure adequate vascularization of the surgical papillae of the coronally advanced flap.

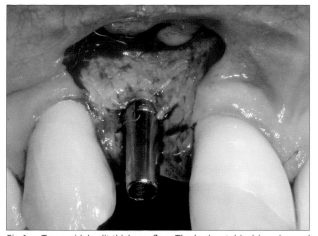

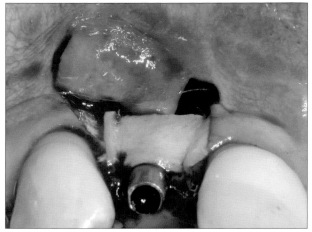

Fig 1e Trapezoidal split-thickness flap. The horizontal incisions (around 3 mm long) were performed apically to the vertex of the anatomic papillae at a distance equivalent to the desired coronal advancement of the flap; the vertical releasing incisions were slightly divergent, reaching into the alveolar mucosa. Deep and superficial split-thickness incisions were performed to allow the coronal advancement of the flap. The de-epithelialization of the anatomic papillae was extended toward the palatal aspect.

Fig 1f Connective-tissue graft derived from the de-epithelialization of a free gingival graft, secured in place at the level of the gingival margin of the adjacent teeth. Graft fixation was performed using internal mattress sutures at the base of the anatomical papillae and external mattress sutures at the apical aspect.

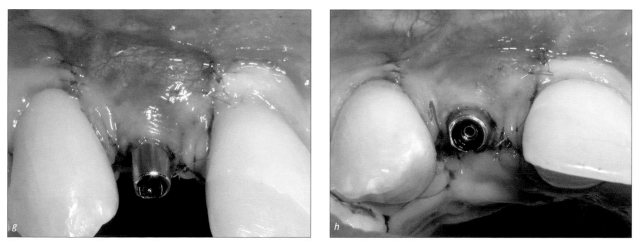

Figs 1g-h The coronally advanced flap was closed, starting at the level of the vertical releasing incisions, using single interrupted sutures and sling sutures, suspended around the cingulum of the adjacent teeth for tight adaptation of the soft-tissue margin around the convexity of the abutment. The connective-tissue graft was completely covered by the flap. A short provisional crown was placed, preventing contact with the soft tissues.

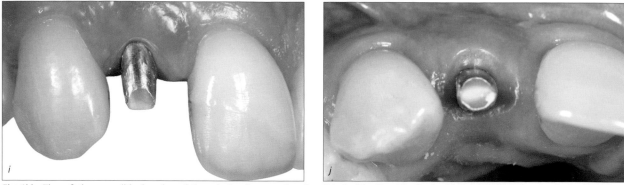

Figs 1i-j   *The soft-tissue conditioning phase followed after four months of undisturbed healing. The final goal was to scallop the marginal soft tissue to make it as similar as possible to the gingival margin of the natural homologous tooth and to promote the coronal growth of the papillae through modifications of the interproximal profiles of the provisional crown.*

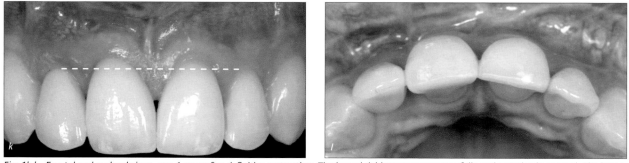

Figs 1k-l   *Frontal and occlusal views, one 1 year after definitive restoration. The buccal dehiscence was successfully and completely covered. The buccolingual increase in soft-tissue volume enabled the creation of a prosthetic crown with a natural emergence profile that resembled those of the adjacent teeth, making the site easier to maintain from a hygienic point of view.*

Several steps are considered essential for the success of this type of treatment, beginning with the removal of the prosthetic crown at least one month before surgery. Short provisional crowns that are not in contact with marginal soft tissue are placed following abutment reduction for undisturbed interproximal soft-tissue growth and maturation.

All defects are treated with a coronally advanced flap (CAF) and a CTG (Zucchelli and coworkers 2003). The flap is elevated as a split-thickness flap. All muscle insertions are eliminated to permit coronal advancement. Any exposed implant surface is mechanically finished using diamond burs and rubber cups. The facial and occlusal portions of the anatomical papillae are de-epithelialized to create connective-tissue beds onto which the surgical papillae of the coronally advanced flap are secured by suturing. The CTG is harvested from the palate as a free gingival graft, and the epithelium is removed with

a sharp blade (Zucchelli and coworkers 2010). The thickness of the free gingival graft is about 2 mm, with a mesiodistal dimension 6 mm greater than the width of the dehiscence defect and an apicocoronal dimension 3 mm greater than the depth of the bone dehiscence.

The graft is positioned to cover the abutment and secured using two resorbable interrupted sutures at the base of the anatomical papillae and two single sutures anchored to the periosteum at the apical aspect.

The flap is mobilized until the soft-tissue margin passively extends to a level coronal to the CTG. The flap is sutured using 6-0 Vicryl in a coronal position to cover the CTG without creating tension. After the surgery, the provisional crown is reduced to avoid contact with the soft tissue and is secured with temporary cement. The sutures are kept in place for two weeks. Patients are instructed not disturb the treated area and to rinse with a

0.12% chlorhexidine solution three times a day for 1 min over four weeks.

After this time, patients are advised to use an ultra-soft toothbrush and a roll technique for one month. During this period, the chlorhexidine rinse is used twice a day. Then, patients are instructed to use a soft toothbrush and rinse with chlorhexidine once a day for another month. When chlorhexidine is discontinued, full mechanical interproximal cleaning in the surgical area is reinstituted. The patients are recalled for prophylaxis every two weeks after suture removal for the first two months and, subsequently, once a month until the final restoration.

Eight months after the surgical procedure, a definitive impression is taken, and the resulting cast is used for abutment selection and crown design. The final shape of the abutment is selected according to the axis of the implant and the soft tissue around it.

Paniz and Mazzocco (2015) described a combined surgical-prosthetic approach to treat a patient's anterior sextant, with a 2-mm recession of the facial soft tissue of an implant, based on the observation that the customization of the prosthetic emergence profile contributes significantly to the final esthetic outcome of the soft tissue. Two surgical procedures were performed, combined with a modification of the prosthetic profile of the provisional restoration and the definitive abutment.

The first surgery was performed after removing the implant restoration and after the peri-implant soft tissue had matured. It employed a CTG and a coronally advanced flap to submerge the implant. The second CTG was inserted into a buccal pouch, and an undercontoured provisional restoration was delivered. The definitive prosthetic phase of treatment followed six months later.

According to the authors, the final esthetic outcome satisfied the patient and resolved the main complaint, remaining stable for five years. It ought to be mentioned that this approach was possible only because the definitive restoration included not only a new customized implant abutment and a crown, but also a crown on the adjacent natural tooth, which provided support for the provisional restoration while the implant was completely submerged.

Surgical techniques only

The first prospective cohort study was presented by Burkhardt and coworkers (2008). Ten patients were treated, each with a single mucosal soft-tissue dehiscence at an implant site. The implants had been inserted according to a delayed protocol, eight of them in a two-stage approach (Nobel Biocare, Zurich, Switzerland; Friadent, Mannheim, Germany) and two (Institut Straumann AG, Basel, Switzerland) in a one-stage approach. Each site presented with an apical displacement of the soft-tissue margin after more than one year of an esthetically pleasing outcome.

The surgical procedure is a modification of the technique described by Allen and Miller (1989). Beginning with an intracrevicular incision on the buccal side of the implant, a partial-thickness mucosal flap is mobilized beyond the mucogingival line after releasing the flap with two vertical incisions, mesially and distally to the recession. The facial portions of the papillae between tooth and implant sites are de-epithelialized to allow coronal repositioning of the flap. A free CTG is taken from the palate in the region of the premolars to first molars using the single incision technique (Lorenzana and Allen 2000). The harvested graft has a thickness of 1.5 to 2 mm; the incision at the donor site is closed with sling sutures. The graft is placed over the implant/abutment junction and adjacent connective-tissue bed at the prepared recipient sites and secured with a resorbable 7-0 suture.

The graft is then covered with the coronally advanced mucosal flap. The mucosal margin is advanced and secured at least 2 mm coronally to the landmark measured at the contralateral tooth reflecting the clinical crown length, by means of 7-0 sling sutures. The sutures are removed only five days after the surgical treatment. Plaque control in the surgically treated area is maintained by means of chlorhexidine for a further two weeks. After this period, the patients are instructed in mechanical tooth cleaning of the treated region using an ultra-soft toothbrush and a roll technique.

Patients are recalled for prophylaxis and follow-up at one, three, and six months. The mean soft-tissue dehiscence coverage was 75% at one month, 70% at three months, and 66% at six months. The authors concluded that the implant sites revealed a substantial and clinically significant improvement, but complete coverage of the peri-implant soft-tissue dehiscence was not achieved at any of the sites.

A modification of this technique was presented by Roccuzzo and coworkers (2014b). It was performed on patients with a shallow soft-tissue dehiscence around non-submerged Tissue Level implants with smooth collars of two different lengths: S (2.8 mm) or SP (1.8 mm) implants (Institut Straumann AG, Basel, Switzerland) (Figs 2 a-h). The thick gingival tissue of the maxillary tuberosity area is preferred as the donor site. After local anesthesia of the recipient and donor sites, an intracrevicular incision is performed, and a partial-thickness

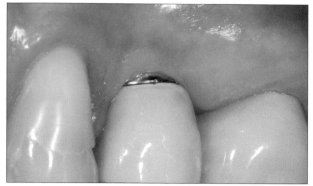

Fig 2a   Peri-implant soft-tissue dehiscence around a Tissue Level implant placed eight years before.

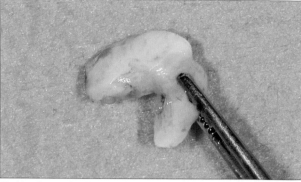

Fig 2b   Connective-tissue grafts taken from the maxillary tuberosity and U-shaped.

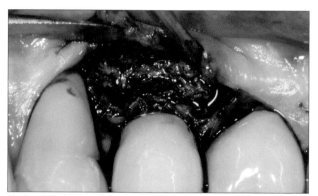

Fig 2c   Split-thickness flap with no releasing vertical incisions.

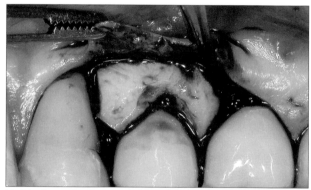

Fig 2d   Connective-tissue graft adapted around the collar of the implant.

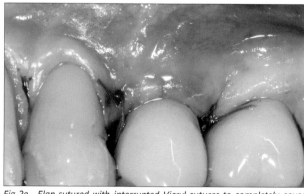

Fig 2e   Flap sutured with interrupted Vicryl sutures to completely cover the CTG.

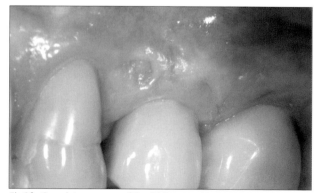

Fig 2f   Complete coverage of the dehiscence at two years.

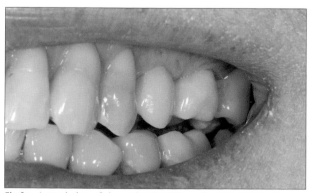

Fig 2g   Lateral view of the patient's smile at six years. The increase in soft-tissue thickness, particularly around the papillae, has resulted in a significant esthetic improvement.

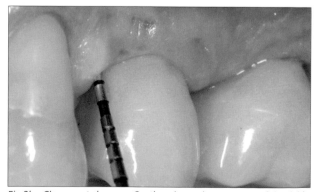

Fig 2h   Close-up at six years. Continued complete coverage of the dehiscence, with minimal probing depth.

flap is elevated. After preparing the recipient site, a gingival cuff-shaped graft is excised from the tuberosity area by a gingivectomy (Jung and coworkers 2008b). The donor tissue is de-epithelialized and trimmed with a mucotome to create a U-shape, to facilitate adaptation to the implant collar. The prepared connective tissue is placed in the recipient bed and immobilized by 6-0 Vicryl sutures (Ethicon; Johnson & Johnson, OH, USA). The flap is secured by 5-0 Vicryl sutures, covering the graft with minimal tension. To achieve this, the muscle insertions are eliminated to allow for coronal advancement. Sutures are kept in place for ten days to two weeks days. Patients are recalled for check-ups and postoperative care as needed. Sometimes a gingivoplasty will be performed after four to eight months, if needed, using a rotating diamond instrument to reduce any excessive bulk and eliminate any color mismatch.

There are three major differences between the Burkhardt and the Roccuzzo approach:

- Vertical incisions were avoided.
- The graft was taken from the maxillary tuberosity.
- The sutures were kept in place more than twice as long.

Figures 3a-i show an example of this treatment approach in a molar area. The soft-tissue dehiscence was a consequence of surgical treatment for peri-implantitis.

Another important open point is whether a minimally invasive treatment of soft-tissue deficiencies around an implant-supported restoration in the esthetic zone can produce good or better results.

The treatment proposed by Cosyn and coworkers (2013) included a CTG harvested from the palate and inserted in the buccal peri-implant mucosa via the envelope (pouch) technique. Hence, this was a prospective study to document soft-tissue aspects for immediate implant treatment following single-tooth extraction. At three months, 5 out 22 cases demonstrated major alveolar process remodeling and 2 showed advanced midfacial recessions. Hence, CTG was performed before delivery of the permanent crown, precluding comparison with the other studies. The authors concluded that to preserve the pink esthetics, CTG may be necessary after immediate implant treatment in about one-third of patients.

Caplanis and coworkers (2014), presenting mucogingival considerations around teeth and implants, illustrated a case with mucosal recession around an implant in the maxillary left canine position exposing approximately 3 mm of the titanium abutment. An envelope flap was elevated with placement of an interpositional CTG harvested from the palate, achieving complete coverage of the exposed titanium abutment in a single surgical procedure. However, for another implant with a mucosal recession exposing 2 mm of the abutment in a central incisor position, three separate surgical procedures were performed to achieve recession coverage: a coronally advanced flap with an interpositional CTG followed by an envelope flap with another interpositional CTG and finally a semi-lunar advanced pedicle flap. The authors concluded that recession repair around implants, as opposed to teeth, is not as well studied or understood, and the treatment is not as predictable.

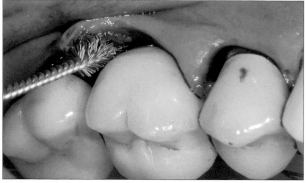

Fig 3a   Surgical treatment of peri-implantitis at site 16 using a titanium brush.

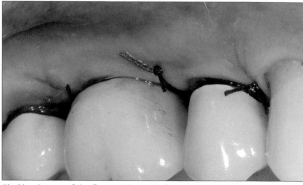

Fig 3b   Suture of the flaps at the end of treatment.

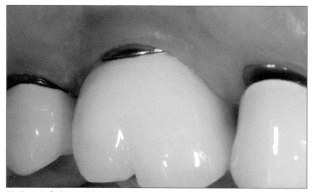

Fig 3c   Soft-tissue dehiscence after surgical treatment of peri-implantitis.

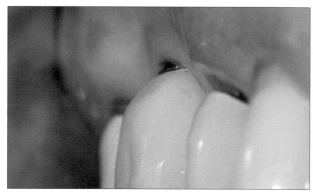

Fig 3d   Lateral view of the soft-tissue dehiscence.

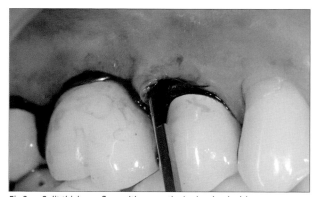

Fig 3e   Split-thickness flap, with no vertical releasing incisions.

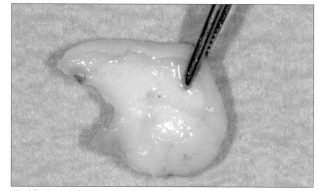

Fig 3f   Connective-tissue graft taken from the tuberosity and made into the shape of a U.

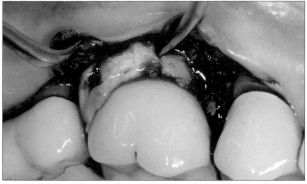

Fig 3g   Adapting the CTG around the collar of the implant.

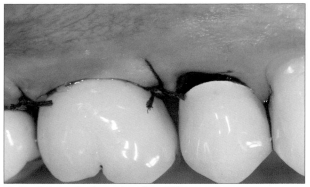

Fig 3h   Suturing the flap on top of the CTG.

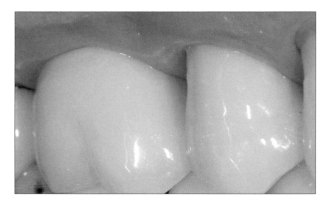

Fig 3i   Optimal healing at two years. A new ceramic crown was placed on the adjacent premolar.

Lee and coworkers (2015) reported one case in a patient presenting with a deficiency in both the horizontal and vertical soft-tissue dimensions around a single-tooth implanted-supported restoration in the anterior maxilla. The soft-tissue defects were augmented with a CTG placed underneath the buccal peri-implant tissue using a frenum-access incision and a supraperiosteal tunneling approach (modified vestibular incision supraperiosteal tunnel access [VISTA] technique, originally described by Zadeh in 2011). According to the authors, this novel technique resulted in an increase in tissue height and width, which suggests its potential use around implant-supported restorations.

It must be noted that all the treatments presented in the literature are in an esthetic area of the maxilla.

Figures 4a-h show an example of this treatment approach in a mandibular area. The soft-tissue dehiscence was limited to about 1 mm, but the patient was not happy with the esthetic result and requested treatment.

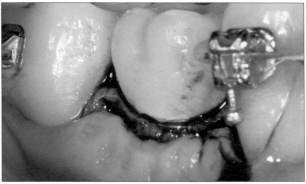

Fig 4a   Tissue Level implant 46 after orthodontic treatment to open the space.

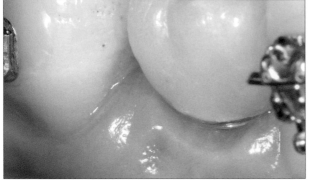

Fig 4b   Split-thickness flap elevated buccally, with no vertical incision, keeping the anatomic papillae intact for close adaptation of the flap.

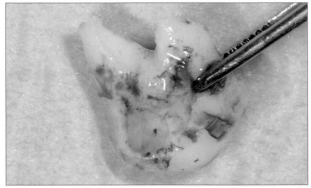

Fig 4c   Large soft-tissue graft harvested from the maxillary tuberosity; epithelium removed with a blade.

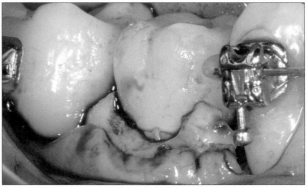

Fig 4d   Placing the connective tissue in the prepared mucoperiosteal envelope, around the collar of the implant.

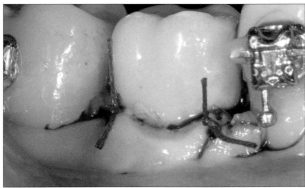

Fig 4e   Flap coronally secured with interrupted 4-0 Vicryl sutures to completely cover the CTG.

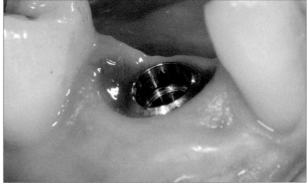

Fig 4f   Status at the time of delivery of the screw-retained ceramic crown.

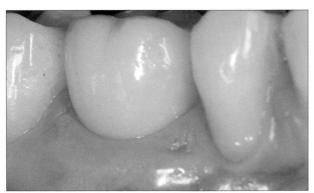

Fig 4g   Buccal view at one year.

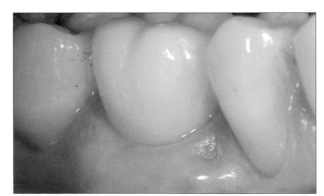

Fig 4h   Buccal view at four years.

Multiple treatments

As the quantity of available connective tissue is often limited, a two-step procedure cannot be excluded if the first treatment does not achieve full coverage. Hidaka and Ueno (2012) presented a case with 3 mm of abutment exposure on an implant replacing tooth 21. The mucosal recession was corrected with a two-stage surgical approach. A partial-thickness pouch was constructed around the dehiscence. A subepithelial CTG was placed and secured by a 7-0 nylon suture in apical position. After covering the graft with a mucosal flap, the flap was coronally advanced and secured with a 7-0 nylon suture. At twelve months, the recipient site was partially covered by keratinized mucosa. However, the buccal interdental papilla between the implant and adjacent lateral incisor was concave in shape. To resolve the mucosal recession after the first graft, a second graft was performed using the same technique. The authors reported that an esthetically satisfactory result was achieved and that the marginal soft-tissue level was stable nine months after the second graft.

It is reasonable to imagine that if the implant/abutment assembly is trimmed, the need for a two-stage procedure may be reduced. However, this must be carefully balanced against the possibility of reducing the resistance of the implant/abutment to fatigue fracture.

Figures 5a-m show an example of a treatment where two procedures were necessary to obtain complete dehiscence coverage.

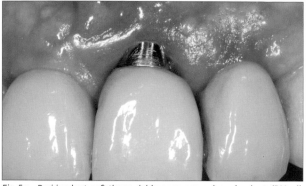

Fig 5a   Peri-implant soft-tissue dehiscence around an implant (RN, diameter 4.1 mm, length 10 mm; Institut Straumann AG), five years after placement.

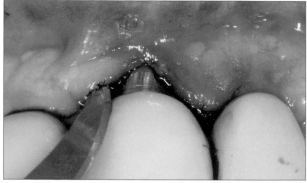

Fig 5b   Trapezoidal split-thickness flap; slightly divergent vertical releasing incisions up to the alveolar mucosa. A 12b blade was used to make the first horizontal incision.

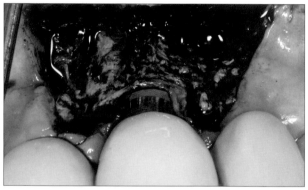

Fig 5c   The exposed implant surface was treated with 24% EDTA (Prefgel, Institut Straumann AG) for two minutes and 1% chlorhexidine gel (Corsodyl dental gel; GlaxoSmithKline, Baranzate, Italy) for another two minutes. It was then thoroughly rinsed with sterile physiologic saline solution, but not mechanically altered. Afterwards, the anatomic papillae were completely de-epithelialized.

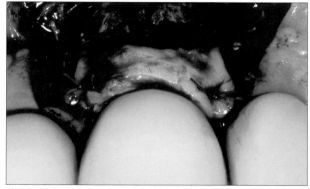

Fig 5d   CTG adapted and sutured with 6-0 Vicryl.

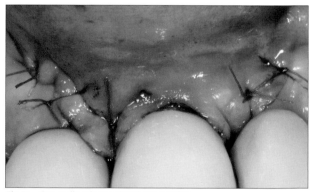

Fig 5e   Coronally advanced and sutured flap.

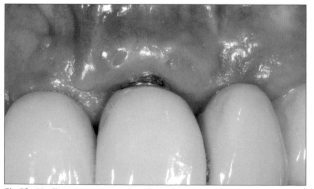

Fig 5f   Healing at seven months. The soft-tissue dehiscence was reduced, but complete coverage was not achieved.

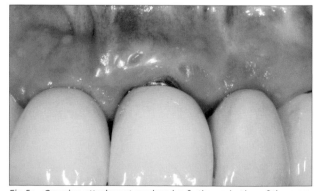

Fig 5g   Creeping attachment produced a further reduction of the recession, two years after the first surgery. Since the patient had high esthetic expectations, a second surgery was proposed.

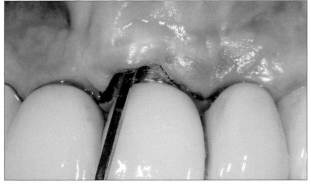

Fig 5h   Split-thickness flap.

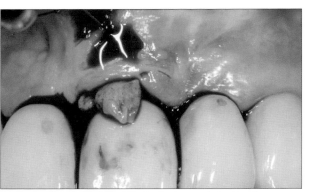

Fig 5i   CTG inserted facially at the implant-supported restoration.

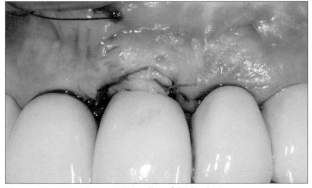

Fig 5j   CTG secured around the collar of the implant.

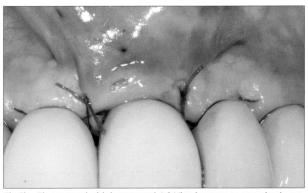

Fig 5k   Flap secured with interrupted 4-0 Vicryl sutures to completely cover the CTG.

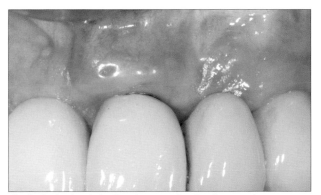

Fig 5l   Optimal early healing three months after the second surgery

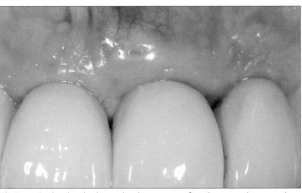

Fig 5m   Optimal esthetic results three years after the second surgery (seven years after baseline). Complete coverage, tissue maturation and stabilization were obtained.

Alternatives to connective-tissue grafts

In recent years, researchers have worked intensively to find a soft-tissue graft substitute that would generate keratinized tissue and increase soft-tissue thickness to eliminate donor site morbidity, ideally available in unlimited quantities off the shelf.

Among the products available in several countries, an acellular dermal matrix graft (ADM) has been proposed as an alternative for gingival recession coverage.

Mareque-Bueno (2011) illustrated the use of an ADM in association with a novel technique of a coronally advanced flap to treat a 3-mm soft-tissue recession on the buccal aspect of a maxillary lateral incisor implant. Triangular-shaped incisions were performed mesially and distally to the implant. The coronal part of the incision was designed as a butt joint and the apical part was beveled. The flap was elevated as a split-thickness flap so that it could be moved coronally over the ADM after de-epithelialization of the triangular area between the incisions. The ADM was trimmed to size and placed in the defect at a level just below the coronal margin of the triangular-shaped incision. The flap and the graft were secured in place using 6-0 polypropylene interrupted sutures. A vertical mattress suture was then provided to hold the flap in a more coronal position. The sutures were removed after two weeks of healing. Six months later, only partial defect coverage had been achieved, even in a case where the recession did not exceed 3 mm; probing depth was 2 mm on the facial aspect, with adequate keratinized gingiva present in the treated area. Even though the author reported that the patient was satisfied with the overall treatment result, some observers may have reservations regarding the overall benefit of the procedure.

Anderson and coworkers (2014) published a randomized controlled clinical pilot trial comparing a subepithelial connective-tissue graft (SCTG) to ADM, both under coronally positioned flaps, in 13 patients presenting with implants displaying recession, thin tissue phenotype, concavity defects, or a combination thereof, associated with single-crown dental implants. Both groups achieved gains in tissue thickness (SCTG, 63%; ADM, 105%), reduced concavity measures (SCTG, 82%; ADM, 96%), and increased recession coverage (SCTG, 40%; ADM, 28%) from baseline to six months. Clinicians determined improvements in esthetics for both groups, unlike patients who did not change their esthetic ratings. ADM subjects had more eventful wound healing. While the authors concluded that both SCTG and ADM have the potential to reduce recessions on definitively restored dental implants, these results should be interpreted with caution,

given the small sample size and the many parameters investigated.

In a recent multicenter pilot study, Schallhorn and coworkers (2015) presented a surgical procedure using porcine collagen matrix where 35 implant sites were treated in 30 patients presenting with gray show-through or contour deficiencies/concavities or with < 2 mm width of keratinized tissue. A gingival pouch was created on the buccal aspect of implant sites utilizing sulcular incisions extending one-half to one full tooth beyond the implant, and a split-thickness flap was reflected. The collagen matrix was trimmed, placed as an interpositional graft on the buccal aspect of implant sites, and if possible secured either by a sling suture or by suturing it to the lingual tissue. At six months, the results indicated that the collagen matrix increased tissue thickness and provided more keratinized tissue around existing dental implants, but results between implants were very variable. While statistically significant gains in gingival thickness and keratinized tissue were observed, no significant changes in gray show-through or soft-tissue contour were found. Even though the authors encouraged additional research to confirm and expand the results of the case series, it is hard to believe this porcine collagen matrix will have a significant role as substitute for a connective-tissue graft.

Treatment of adjacent sites
All cases presented in the literature are, to the best of our knowledge, limited to single recessions. Figures 6a-k present a case of a female patient with a recession involving two adjacent tissue-level implants.

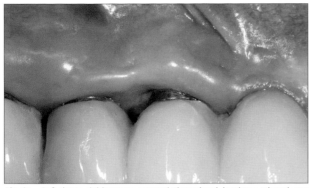

Fig 6a   Soft-tissue dehiscences around tissue-level implants placed one year before.

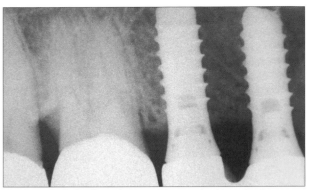

Fig 6b   Periapical radiograph. Normal interproximal bone levels.

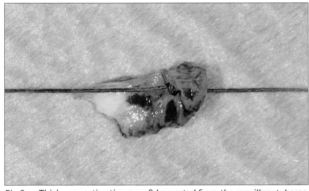

Fig 6c   Following a horizontal incision beyond the mucogingival line, a subperiosteal tunnel was created extending one tooth to the mesial and one tooth to the distal.

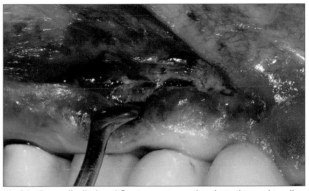

Fig 6d   Coronally displaced flap to create a subperiosteal tunnel to allow for tension-free coronal repositioning of the margin.

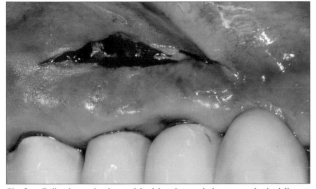

Fig 6e   Thick connective-tissue graft harvested from the maxillary tuberosity, fixed to a resorbable suture.

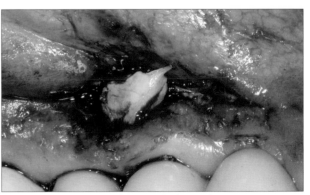

Fig 6f   Connective-tissue graft inserted in the pouch.

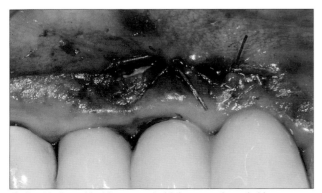

Fig 6g   Horizontal incision secured with interrupted resorbable sutures.

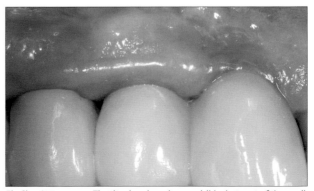

Fig 6h   At two years. The titanium is no longer visible, but part of the papilla is still missing. Plaque control is not ideal, particularly in the cantilever region. Patient is motivated and re-instructed for proper home hygiene care.

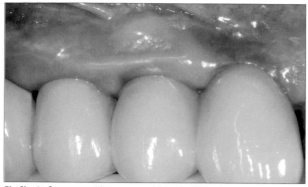

Fig 6i   At four years. Plaque control has significantly improved, and the papilla has completely filled the space between the two implants.

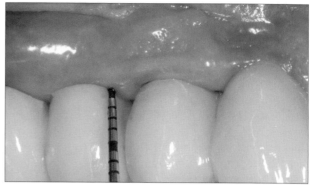

Fig 6j   At five years. Soft tissue remains stable and healthy, with minimal probing depth and no bleeding.

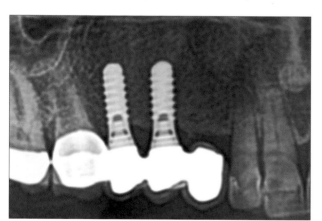

Fig 6k   Panoramic radiograph. Normal interproximal bone level at nine years.

Free gingival grafts

While the use of free gingival grafts seems to be indicated when there is a need to increase the vestibular depth, to remove an aberrant frenum, or to reduce soreness during oral hygiene procedures, as indicated by Roccuzzo and coworkers (2016), it does not seem the most effective technique for peri-implant soft-tissue dehiscence coverage. This has already been thoroughly described in Chapter 4.1.

At the time of publication, one study was extant to describe the coverage of a soft-tissue dehiscence around a single implant with a free gingival graft. Fickl (2015) presented the use of such a graft for a shallow peri-implant mucosal recession around a lower incisor implant in an area with a lack of attached keratinized mucosa. After apical repositioning of the mucogingival border and decontamination of the implant, a free gingival graft was successfully stabilized to cover the implant dehiscence. The author stated that "the predictability of completely covering peri-implant mucosal recessions is low. Shallow (1 to 2 mm) recession-type defects around implants seem manageable with a coronally repositioned flap and subepithelial connective-tissue grafts." Indeed, the second case presented in the paper is a shallow peri-implant mucosal recession buccal to a right upper lateral incisor, treated with a coronally repositioned flap and a connective-tissue graft.

An alternative approach: guided bone regeneration

In a retrospective clinical case series, Le and coworkers (2016) first presented the treatment of soft-tissue dehiscence at implant sites in the esthetic zone using a guided bone regeneration (GBR) approach. The rationale is based on the idea that gingival/mucosal height is influenced by the position of the underlying bone, and that peri-implant bone loss can result in soft-tissue recession.

Only patients with bone loss confined to the labial surface of the implant were selected. They were treated with a GBR protocol to resolve bone defects. After crown removal and placement of a healing abutment, a crestal incision and a distal curvilinear vertical incision were made that followed the gingival margin of the distal proximal tooth. A full-thickness subperiosteal flap was elevated on the labial aspect of the implant to expose a field two to three times the size of treatment area, and the papilla was reflected on the mesial side of the implant site. Tissue was removed from the osseous defect using a curette, and the site was irrigated to remove debris. The peri-implant soft tissue was released and advanced by scoring the periosteum so that tension free closure could be achieved. A mineralized allograft and a resorbable membrane were used in a GBR surgical procedure, in combination with a roughened titanium tenting screw placed 3 to 4 mm below the implant platform to restore unesthetic defects in the anterior maxilla.

After four months of non-submerged healing, a screw-retained provisional prosthesis was made, with the definitive restoration being delivered four to five months later. One year after treatment, the mean mid-implant buccal bone thickness had increased by 1.84 mm. Significant mean increases of 1.28, 1.29, and 1.23 mm in soft-tissue thickness, keratinized tissue width, and gingival height, respectively, were also noted. The authors concluded that the use of the allograft and xenogeneic membrane effectively increased alveolar hard and soft-tissue dimensions in the esthetic zone of the anterior maxilla.

Long-term results

Zucchelli and coworkers (2019) were the first authors to report five-year clinical and esthetic outcomes of a novel surgical/prosthetic approach for the treatment of buccal soft-tissue dehiscences around single dental implants. Twenty patients with buccal soft-tissue dehiscence around single implants in the esthetic zone were treated by removing the implant-supported crown, reducing the implant abutment, reflecting a coronally advanced flap in combination with a connective-tissue graft, and delivering a prosthetic restoration. After the first year, patients were recalled three times a year until the final clinical re-evaluation five years after the final prosthetic crown. Of the 20 patients enrolled in the study, 19 completed it after five years. A total of 99.2% mean soft-tissue dehiscence coverage, with 79% of complete dehiscence coverage, was achieved after these five years. A statistically significant increase in buccal soft-tissue thickness and keratinized tissue height was demonstrated at five years compared to one year. The esthetic evaluation showed high visual analog scale (VAS) scores with no statistical difference between one year and five years. A statistic significant improvement in pink/white esthetic scores (PES/WES) was observed between baseline and five years, but not between one and five years. The authors concluded that successful esthetic and soft-tissue dehiscence coverage outcomes were well maintained at five years. The strict regime of postsurgical control visits and the emphasis placed on controlling of the toothbrushing technique could have been critical for the successful long-term maintenance of soft-tissue dehiscence coverage results.

More recently, Roccuzzo and coworkers (2019) reported five-year outcomes covering shallow maxillary soft-tissue dehiscences around single tissue-level implants. The original population consisted of 16 patients presenting with soft-tissue recession at a single maxillary buccal implant. A connective-tissue graft, taken from the maxillary tuberosity, was placed underneath a split-thickness envelope flap. After treatment, the patients received individual supportive periodontal therapy. Two patients were lost to follow-up; one implant was removed due to peri-implantitis before the final examination. At five years, complete soft-tissue coverage of the implants was observed in 8 of 13 cases (62%). Mean soft-tissue dehiscence coverage was 86%. The patients' esthetic evaluation showed persistent high VAS scores. The authors concluded that the treatment of buccal soft-tissue dehiscences around single implants, followed by regular supportive therapy, yielded good esthetic and functional results in the majority of patients.

Acknowledgments

Clinical procedures (Fig 1)
Prof. Giovanni Zucchelli, Dr. Martina Stefanini – University of Bologna, Italy

Prosthetic procedures (Fig 1)
Dr. Giuseppe Pellitteri – Bolzano, Italy

Laboratory procedures (Figs 2 – 6)
Francesco Cataldi – Torino, Italy

5.2.1   Tunneling Technique for Treating Peri-Implant Soft-Tissue Dehiscences

A. Sculean

Emerging evidence indicates that various modifications of the tunneling technique can be successfully used to treat single and multiple mandibular and maxillary gingival recessions (Aroca and coworkers 2010, 2013; Sculean and coworkers 2014b, 2016, 2017a, 2017b; Sculean and Allen 2018).

Novel modifications of the tunnel technique—the modified coronally advanced tunnel (MCAT) and the laterally closed tunnel (LCT) consisting of a combined full-thickness and partial-thickness pouch or tunnel/flap followed by coronal or lateral displacement—have demonstrated excellent outcomes in various locations, including very deep mandibular recessions. (Sculean and coworkers 2014b, 2016, 2017a, 2017b; Sculean and Allen 2018).

MCAT and LCT provide the following advantages:

*   No or minimal need to perform vertical releasing incisions and keep the papillae intact, thus facilitating vascularization of the area and stabilizing the tunneled flap.
*   Predictable coverage of soft-tissue dehiscences through coronal or lateral displacement of the tunneled flap to completely cover and protect the soft-tissue graft.

It has also been shown that MCAT in conjunction with a subepithelial connective-tissue graft (SCTG) yielded excellent coverage of single and multiple gingival recessions at teeth restored with crowns in the maxillary esthetic zone, minimizing or in most cases eliminating the need to replace the restorations (Sculean and coworkers 2017).

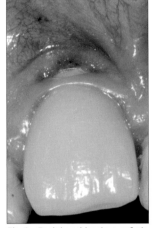

Fig 1   *Facial peri-implant soft-tissue dehiscence affecting esthetics and cleansability.*

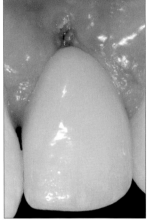

Fig 2   *Facial peri-implant soft-tissue dehiscence affecting esthetics and cleansability. Lack of attached keratinized mucosa at the dehiscence site.*

MCAT and LCT can be also used to treat small (2 – 3 mm) peri-implant soft-tissue dehiscences in cases where the implant is positioned in an acceptable orofacial position, with its greatest part located within the bony envelope, and without signs of peri-implantitis (Figs 1 and 2) (Sculean and coworkers 2017a).

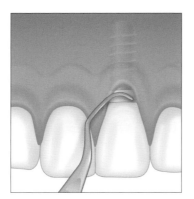

Fig 3 Cleaning the exposed implant surface with a titanium curette.

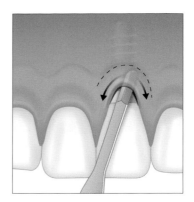

Fig 4 Intrasulcular incision to facilitate subsequent vertical penetration of the tunneling knife.

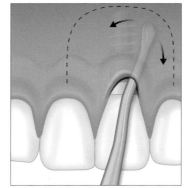

Fig 5 Full-thickness preparation of the tunnel through careful vertical and lateral movement of the tunneling knife.

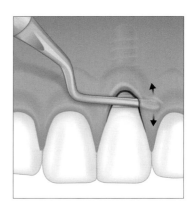

Fig 6 Lateral preparation of the full-thickness tunnel. The preparation extends to the line angle of the adjacent tooth.

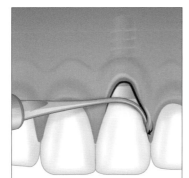

Fig 7 Mobilization of the papilla using a specially designed tunneling knife (Sculean-Aroca) to enable coronal or lateral displacement of the tunnel margins.

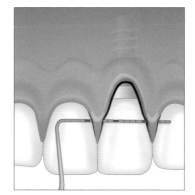

Fig 8 Prepared tunnel. The periodontal probe can pass under the undermined mesial and distal papilla.

The surgical technique for both, MCAT and LCT, consists of the following steps:

- After local anesthesia, the exposed implant surface is cleaned with titanium curettes, air polishing devices using either glycine or erythritol powder, or a combination of the two (Fig 3).
- Intrasulcular incisions using microsurgical blades are made in the sulcular area in order to facilitate

the penetration of tunneling knives into the submucosal area to prepare a full-thickness tunnel (Fig 4). The tunneled flap is prepared vertically beyond the mucogingival junction and extended mesially and distally, undermining the adjacent interdental papillae but leaving them intact (Figs 5 to 9).

- If deemed necessary, the frenula, muscles fibers or inserting fibers from the inner aspect of the flap are removed using microsurgical blades or conventional

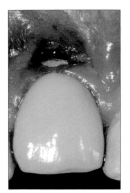

Fig 9   The prepared tunnel (case depicted in Fig 1).

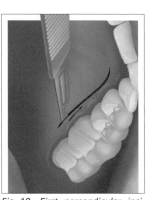

Fig 10   First perpendicular incision to the palate with a #15 or #15c blade.

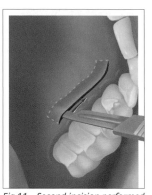

Fig 11   Second incision performed parallel to the palatal epithelium to dissect the underlying connective tissue.

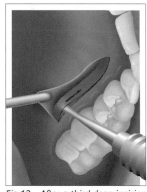

Fig 12   After a third deep incision parallel to the bone, the connective-tissue graft is carefully detached using a periosteal elevator.

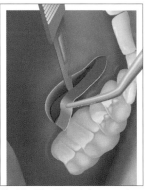

Fig 13   The SCTG is harvested using a #15 or #15c blade.

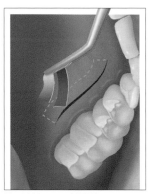

Fig 14 Harvested SCTG.

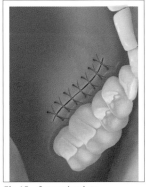

Fig 15   Sutured palate.

#15C surgical blades until tension-free coronal mobilization of the flap is achieved. If needed, the interdental parts of the papillae can be also gently undermined using specially designed tunneling knives (Sculean-Aroca; Stoma, Liptingen, Germany) (Fig 7). However, care must be taken not to disrupt the interdental papillary tissues and to avoid flap perforation.

- After tunnel preparation, a palatal SCTG 1–1.5 mm in thickness is harvested by using the single-incision technique (Figs 10 to 14) (Hürzeler and Weng 1999; Lorenzana and Allen 2000).
- Immediately after harvesting, the donor site is closed with continuous sutures, mattress sutures, suspended sutures, or single interrupted sutures (Fig 15).

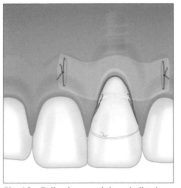

Fig 16 Following mesial and distal accommodation of the SCTG in the tunnel with horizontal mattress sutures. The graft is sutured over the exposed part of the implant using sling sutures.

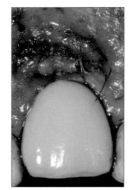

Fig 17 Fixed SCTG over the exposed part of the implant (case depicted in Fig 1).

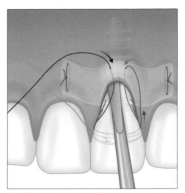

Fig 18 The tunneled flap is moved coronally by a sling suture. Periosteal elevator interposed between the SCTG and the mucosa to avoid contact between the needle and the SCTG.

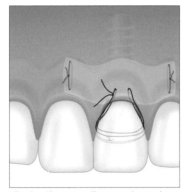

Fig 19 The coronally sutured tunnel covers the SCTG and the mucosal dehiscence.

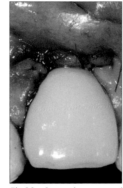

Fig 20 Sutured tunnel (case depicted in Fig 1).

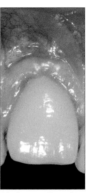

Fig 21 Complete coverage of the mucosal recession (case shown in Fig 1).

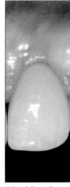

Fig 22 Complete resolution of the mucosal recession (case shown in Fig 2). Significant gain in attached KAM.

- The SCGT is pulled into the tunnel and secured at the inner aspect of the tunneled flap with single or mattress sutures. The graft is attached to the exposed implant surface using sling sutures, with the knot placed orally (Figs 16 and 17).
- Finally, the tunneled flap is either coronally advanced using sling sutures (for the MCAT) or closed laterally with single interrupted sutures (for the LCT), to completely cover the SCTG and the soft-tissue dehiscence (Figs 18 to 20).

The postoperative protocol includes the administration of anti-inflammatory or analgesic medication for two to three days, and optional prescription of systemic antibiotics. Infection control is usually ensured by rinsing with a 0.2%, 0.1%, or 0.12% chlorhexidine digluconate solution twice daily for 1 min during the first two to three weeks postoperatively.

The palatal sutures are removed seven to ten days after surgery, while those from the dehiscence area are removed at two to three weeks. After suture removal, patients are instructed in how to mechanically clean the surgical sites: using an ultra-soft manual toothbrush, patients are asked to employ the roll technique, gradually returning to the regular oral hygiene habits at one month after surgery. Recall appointments including professional supragingival tooth and implant cleaning and individually designed oral hygiene instructions are usually scheduled at one, three, six, and twelve months postoperatively. Clinical outcomes are usually evaluated at six and twelve months (Figs 21 and 22).

6 <u>Clinical Case Presentations</u>

6.1   Implant Placement in the Esthetic Zone and Coverage of Multiple Gingival Recessions

S. Aroca

Presenting complaint

A 47-year-old woman was referred by her general dental practitioner for the treatment of generalized gingival recessions and the extraction of tooth 21 due to external root resorption. The patient had high esthetic expectations. Her main concern was the appearance of the anterior teeth and their "elongation." The patient had no symptoms related to the resorption process on root 21 but had been advised of the condition by her practitioner.

Clinical examination revealed multiple gingival recessions on the facial aspect of the anterior maxillary teeth from 14 to 24, with an otherwise stable periodontal status and good plaque control (GI = 0; PI < 10%) (Table 1; Fig 1).

Cone-beam computed tomography (CBCT) scans confirmed the external resorption of tooth 21. The loss of the facial cortical plate is evident (Figs 2a-b).

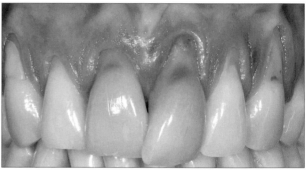

Fig 1   Multiple recessions.

Table 1   Periodontal indices at presentation.

PD	14	13	12	11	21	22	23	24
Mesial	2	2	2	1	2	1	2	3
Distal	2	3	2	2	3	2	2	2

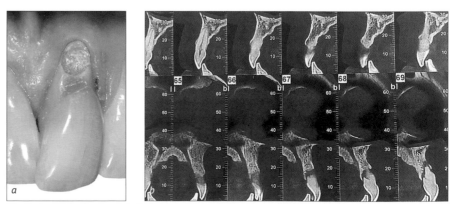

Figs 2a-b   Clinical and radiological view of the external root resorption of tooth 21.

Taking into consideration the patient's high esthetic expectations, the following treatment approach was proposed:

Multiple root coverage extending from tooth 14 to tooth 24 by using the modified tunnel technique (Aroca and coworkers 2013). The patient received detailed explanations on the surgical root coverage using by one of the following two options:

- Connective-tissue graft harvested from the palate
- Soft-tissue augmentation using a collagen matrix as grafting material

After a detailed explanation of the procedures, risks, and benefits, the patient preferred the second option and consented to the surgical procedure.

Treatment procedures

All teeth from 14 to 24 were splinted with composite at the incisal angles to support suspended sutures. During this first phase of the treatment, tooth 21 was retained to facilitate better support for the coronally advanced tunnel (Azzi and Etienne 1998; Aroca and coworkers 2010; Aroca and coworkers 2013) underneath which a trimmed 30 × 40-mm collagen matrix was placed (Mucoderm; Botiss Biomaterials, Zossen, Germany) (Figs 3a-b).

There was a discrepancy of the available mesiodistal gap width at site 21 due to tooth rotation. Six months after the first surgical phase and before the extraction of tooth 21, orthodontic treatment was performed to increase the mesiodistal distance of site 21. The extraction of the upper left incisor was followed by a socket preservation technique according to the GBR principle. The Bio-Gide membrane was briefly placed between the inner surface of the soft-tissue pouch and the buccal bone, ensuring that the size of the membrane exceeded the contour

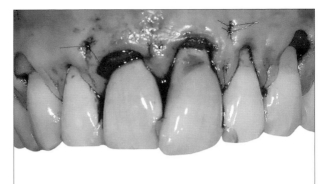

Fig 3a   Collagen matrix placed under the tunnel and fixed by sutures (6-0 prolene and 5-0 polyglactin 910; Ethicon).

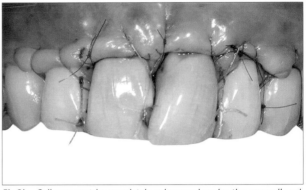

Fig 3b   Collagen matrix completely submerged under the coronally advanced tunnel with suspended sutures around the contact points.

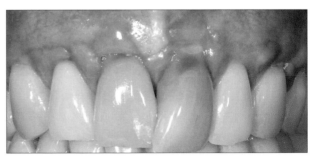

Fig 4   After three weeks of healing.

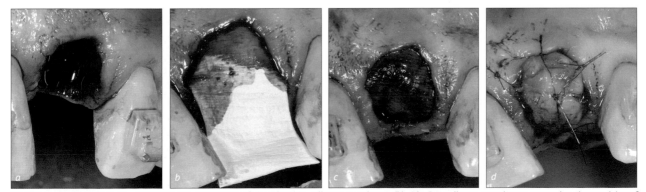

Figs 5a-d   Atraumatic tooth extraction (a). Placement of the Bio-Gide collagen membrane (b). Bio-Oss collagen membrane protecting the particles of deproteinized bovine bone mineral (c). Connective-tissue graft (CTG) sealing the socket (d).

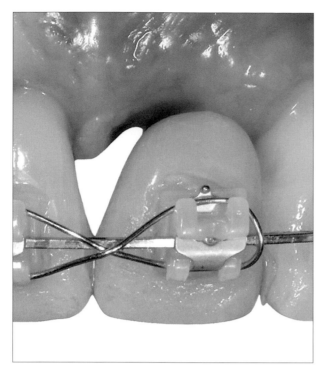

Fig 6 *Clinical situation at three months. The mesiodistal distance at the site of 21 is enlarged.*

of the bony lesion. The socket was filled with particles of deproteinized bovine bone mineral (Bio-Oss and Bio-Gide; Geistlich, Wolhusen, Switzerland) (Figs 5a-d). The socket opening was closed with a connective-tissue graft harvested from the palate using the single-incision technique (Hürzeler and Weng 1999). A single incision was made between the distal aspect of the canine and the mesial aspect of the second molar. An adequate size of the CTG was obtained to seal the socket. The donor site was sutured with modified-horizontal mattress sutures (5-0 polyglactin 910, Vicryl; Ethicon, Johnson & Johnson, New Brunswick, DE, USA).

Six months after the tooth extraction and socket preservation, an implant was placed (RC BLT, diameter 4.1 mm, length 8 mm: Institut Straumann AG, Basel, Switzerland) using a tunnel approach (Aroca and coworkers 2010; Aroca and coworkers 2013) without releasing incisions, and the marginal mucosa was augmented using a connective-tissue graft from the palate (Fig 7).

A provisional crown was fitted immediately upon completion of the surgical procedures. Figures 8a-b show the clinical and radiological situation at three weeks with the provisional crown in place.

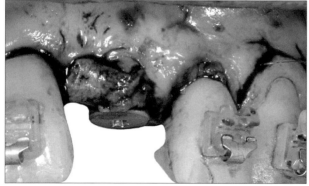

Fig 7 *Simultaneous placement of the implant and connective-tissue using a tunnel approach to support the marginal mucosa.*

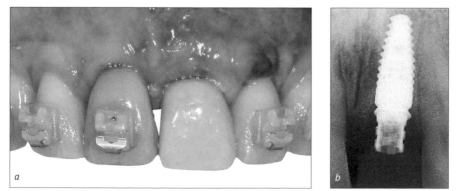

Figs 8a-b *Clinical and radiological view at three weeks with the provisional crown placed immediately after implant placement.*

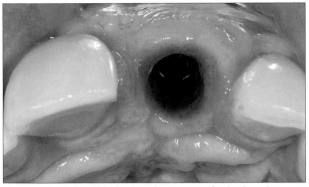

Fig 9   Occlusal view of the implant site one year after implant placement.

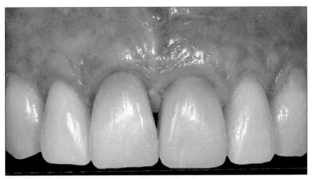

Fig 10   Definitive crown.

All sites of gingival recession remained successfully covered, with stable peri-implant hard and soft tissues 2.5 years after the prosthetic restoration (Figs 11 and 12).

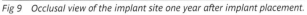

Fig 11   2.5 years after delivery of the restoration.

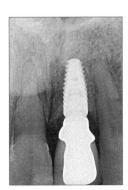

Fig 12   Radiographic view 2.5 years after delivery of the restoration.

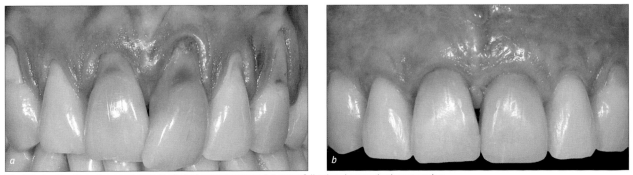

Figs 13a-b   Baseline view compared to clinical appearance at 2.5 years following the prosthetic restoration.

Discussion

The modified tunnel technique is a technique described first by Azzi and Etienne (1998) and Aroca and coworkers (2010; 2013). The "tunnel" flap is created using a full-thickness dissection extended beyond the mucogingival junction and under each papilla, so that the flap can be moved in a coronal direction without tension. Muscle fibers and any remaining collagen bundles on the inner aspect of the mucosal flap are cut using Gracey curettes with extreme care to avoid perforation of the flap and to obtain a passive coronal positioning of the flap and the papilla.

The collagen matrix was then inserted under the modified tunnel at the sites of recession and retracted laterally by sutures towards each end of the tunnel. After positioning the collagen matrix laterally, the site was rinsed with saline solution to remove any clots. Then the flap was coronally repositioned, slightly above the cemento-enamel junction, with suspended sutures around the contact points (Azzi and Etienne 1998; Aroca and coworkers 2010; Aroca and coworkers 2013) (Fig 3b), which allowed complete coverage of the collagen matrix.

This approach has demonstrated to be highly effective in root coverage procedures for Miller class 1, 2, and 3 multiple recession defects (90% and 83%, respectively) (Aroca and coworkers 2010; Aroca and coworkers 2013).

The proposed technique will not only cover the gingival recession, but also augment the tissue across the anterior area, including the planned implant site.

The gingival phenotype (thin vs. thick) is of paramount importance in implant dentistry, especially in the esthetic zones of the mouth, a thick phenotype being associated with a reduced risk for soft-tissue recession following crown delivery (Evans and Chen 2008).

Ridge preservation was performed to enhance the possibility of maintaining the shape and volume of the alveolar area, reducing the effect of bone remodeling following tooth extraction (Mardas and coworkers 2015; MacBeth and coworkers 2017; Avila-Ortiz and coworkers 2019).

6.2 Periodontal Plastic Surgery and Prosthetic Procedures to Treat Peri-Implant Soft-Tissue Dehiscences

P. Casentini

A 30-year-old woman was referred by her general dentist for evaluation of an esthetic complication related to previous implant treatment for congenitally missing maxillary lateral incisors.

The patient's chief complaint was the inadequate esthetic appearance of her smile. She reported that 10 years ago, she had been treated with dental implants for the replacement of the two congenitally missing incisors. Following the initial treatment, the patient was satisfied with the overall treatment outcome, but the esthetic appearance progressively deteriorated over the following years.

Her previous dental history and current condition did not reveal any other significant dental or periodontal pathology in her remaining dentition. The patient was not taking any medication and reported being in good general health. She had realistic esthetic expectations for the outcome of treatment.

The extraoral examination revealed a high smile line, with full exposure of maxillary teeth and surrounding soft tissues up to the first-molar region (Fig 1).

The intraoral examination showed two asymmetric implant-supported cemented crowns on teeth 12 and 22, with exposed implant abutments and discoloration of the peri-implant soft tissues (Fig 2).

The soft-tissue phenotype was classified as thin and highly scalloped, with slight gingival recessions at the adjacent teeth. The peri-implant probing values ranged from 2 to 4 mm, with no bleeding on probing. The patient presented with good oral hygiene with a full-mouth plaque score (FMPS) of less than 15%, and the full-mouth probing chart did not reveal any pockets deeper than 3 to 4 mm.

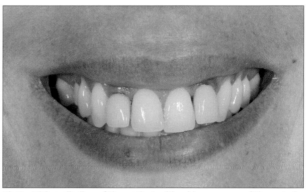

Fig 1   High smile line of the patient with wide exposure of the anterior maxillary teeth.

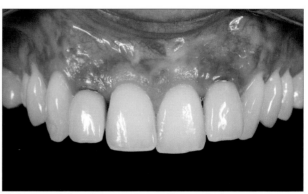

Fig 2   Frontal view of the anterior maxillary teeth: the two implant-supported crowns on tooth 12 and 22 were asymmetric with exposed abutments and discoloration of the surrounding soft tissues.

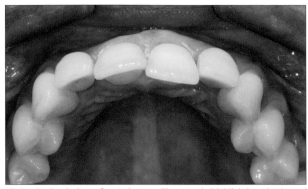

Fig 3   Occlusal view of anterior maxillary teeth highlighting the buccal position of the two crowns.

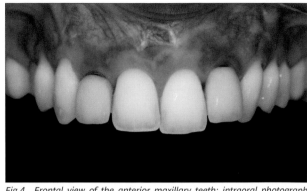

Fig 4   Frontal view of the anterior maxillary teeth: intraoral photograph taken with polarized light highlights the peri-implant soft-tissue discoloration.

The central incisors were misaligned. The occlusal view confirmed mild incisor crowding and an excessively buccal position of the lateral incisor crowns (Fig 3).

An intraoral photograph taken with a polarizing filter confirmed and highlighted the presence of the soft-tissue discoloration at the buccal aspect of the implant crowns (Fig 4).

Intraoral radiographs showed adequate osseointegration of the implants with limited coronal bone remodeling (Figs 5 and 6).

Esthetic analysis

The following issues did not represent an adequate esthetic appearance (Fig 7) when compared to average parameters (Magne and Belser 2002):

- Different shapes of the two lateral incisors; there was an obvious difference in crown length
- Diverging axes of the two lateral incisors rather than being slightly convergent to the midline
- Different soft-tissue levels: in particular, the soft-tissue level at site 12 was too far coronal compared to the adjacent teeth. Conversely, the tissue level at site 22 was too far apical

- The two central incisors had different incisal-edge levels

Treatment planning

Based on the clinical and radiological situation, retention of the existing implants was judged possible and seemed a more convenient option in terms of morbidity and cost. An alternative treatment option would have been the removal of the existing implants and placement of new implants after soft- and hard-tissue augmentation; this was considered too invasive. The following treatment plan was proposed:

- Preliminary orthodontic treatment to relieve crowding and improve the tooth alignment
- Removal of the old crowns and placement of new temporary crowns
- If possible, removal and reshaping of old implant abutments
- Periodontal plastic surgery to increase the thickness of the peri-implant soft tissues and to obtain an optimal position of the peri-implant soft-tissue margins in relation to the future crown, as well as to treat the gingival recessions on the adjacent teeth
- Final prosthetic reconstruction with new ceramic crowns on 12 and 22

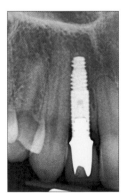

Fig 5   Intraoral radiograph of implant 12.

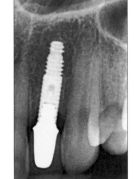

Fig 6   Intraoral radiograph of implant 22.

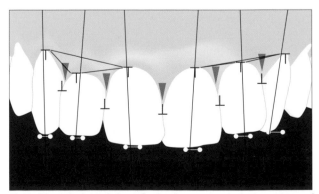

Fig 7   The esthetic analysis confirming the asymmetric shapes and axes of the lateral incisors and asymmetric gingival-margin positions. The incisal edge of the two central incisors is not aligned.

The patient rejected the orthodontic treatment for financial and time reasons and wished to limit the periodontal plastic surgery, if possible, to the implant sites only. She agreed to the rest of the proposed treatment plan and gave her written informed consent.

Preliminary prosthetic procedures
Following the removal of the old crowns (Figs 8 and 9), the abutments were unscrewed and the chamfer finishing line was changed to a vertical edge (Fig 10). This procedure creates more space for the soft tissues and is considered an important step prior to soft-tissue grafting (Zucchelli and coworkers 2013b). Peri-implant probing after abutment removal confirmed the absence of deep pockets and bleeding on probing.

After reconnecting the abutments (Fig 11), two resin temporary crowns were relined with autopolymerizing resin and cemented to the abutments (Fig 12).

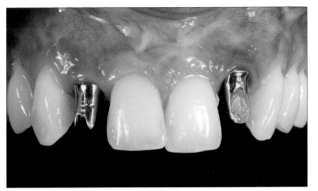

Fig 8   Frontal view after removal of the crowns.

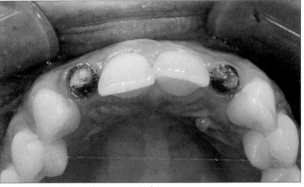

Fig 9   Occlusal view after removal of the crowns.

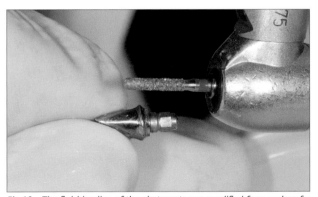

Fig 10   The finishing line of the abutments was modified from a chamfer to a vertical edge.

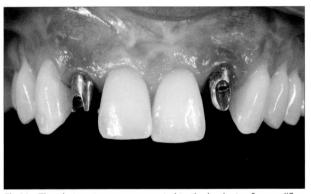

Fig 11   The abutments were reconnected to the implants after modification of the finishing line.

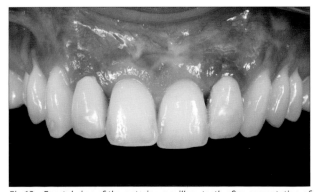

Fig 12   Frontal view of the anterior maxillary teeth after cementation of the temporary crowns 12 and 22.

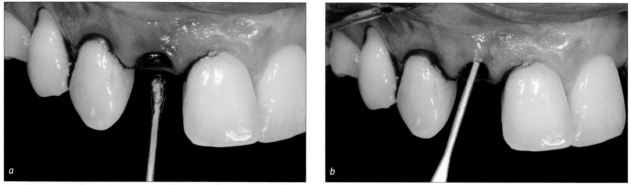

Figs 13a-c   Tunneling technique on site 12: a tunnel was created with a special microsurgical blade.

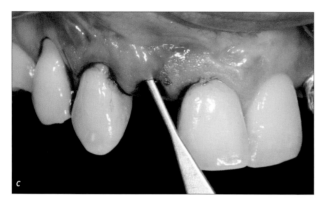

Periodontal plastic surgery

Since the surgical objectives differed between sites 12 and 22, different flap designs were selected for each.

At site 12, there was no need of coronal advancement of the soft-tissue margin; the main goal of surgery was to increase the thickness of the marginal soft tissues. Therefore, it was decided to use a tunneling technique, which is usually less invasive (compared to flap elevation) and results in a faster healing process. Conversely, at site 22, where the surgical objective was coronal advancement of the soft-tissue margin combined with soft-tissue thickening, a coronally advanced flap (CAF) with a connective-tissue graft was selected.

Surgery was performed under local anesthesia in two separate steps.

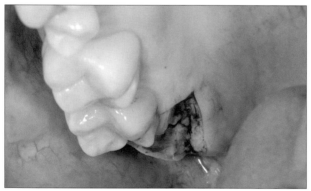

Fig 14   The maxillary tuberosity was used as a donor site.

Site 12. The prosthetic abutment was removed to simplify surgical access. Then a tunnel was created with a microsurgical blade (Spoon Shape 2.0 mm; Omnia, Fidenza, Italy) (Figs 13a-c and 14).

Once the tunnel was created, a connective-tissue graft was harvested from the area of the maxillary tuberosity (Fig 14).

If the tuberosity is available as a donor site, using it has a number of benefits (Roccuzzo and coworkers 2014b), as a high-quality, dense connective-tissue graft without fatty tissue can be harvested here with a reduced risk of postoperative bleeding and without major postoperative pain.

The harvested tissue was subsequently reshaped and de-epithelized with a #15C surgical blade (Fig 15).

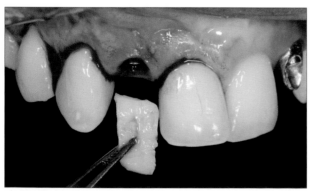

Fig 15   The connective-tissue graft before insertion in the tunnel.

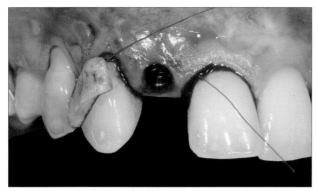

Fig 16 Connective-tissue graft pulled inside the tunnel with sutures.

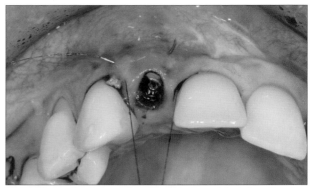

Fig 17 Connective-tissue graft stabilized to the recipient site with a horizontal suture.

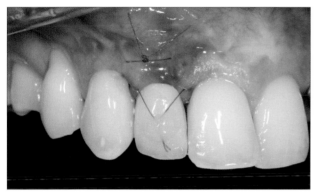

Fig 18 Suspended suture bonded to the temporary crown.

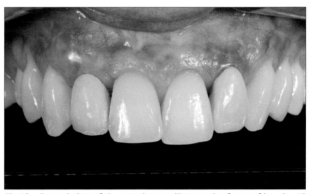

Fig 19 Frontal view of the anterior maxillary teeth after grafting site 12 and before periodontal plastic surgery at site 22.

The graft was then pulled inside the tunnel using 6-0 resorbable polyglycolic-acid sutures (Vicryl Ethicon; Johnson & Johnson Medical, New Brunswick, NJ, USA) (Fig 16). Another suture stabilized the graft horizontally at the recipient site (Fig 17). Finally, after cementation of the temporary crown, the graft was stabilized vertically by a suspended suture bonded to the crown with flowable composite (Fig 18). Chlorhexidine mouth rinses were prescribed for three weeks together with a non-steroidal anti-inflammatory medication for pain relief. The patient was advised to avoid brushing the operation sites for three weeks.

The sutures were removed at two weeks. No complications were recorded, and the patient did not report significant symptoms. Surgery for site 22 was planned after a healing period of six weeks (Fig 19).

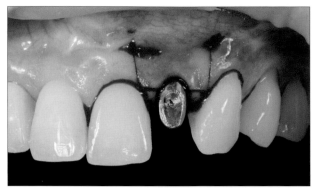

Fig 20   Coronally advanced flap at site 22: flap design.

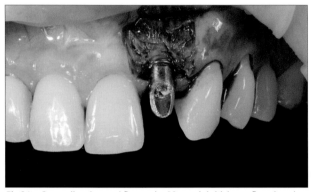

Fig 21   Coronally advanced flap at site 22: partial-thickness flap elevation.

Site 22. After removal of the temporary crown, a trapezoidal partial-thickness flap was elevated to improve the revascularization of the graft. Mesial and distal releasing incisions were extended 2 mm apically to the mucogingival line. The partial-thickness flap was extended over the mucogingival line and the muscle fibers were sectioned to allow coronal advancement of the flap without tension (Figs 20 and 21).

The exposed implant surface (less than 1 mm) was polished with a diamond bur and rinsed with sterile saline and chlorhexidine gel. Subsequently, a connective-tissue graft harvested from the left maxillary tuberosity was de-epithelized and fixed to the buccal periosteum with resorbable 7-0 polyglycolic-acid sutures (PGA; Stoma, Emmingen-Liptingen, Germany) (Figs 22 and 23).

After fixing the connective-tissue graft, the flap was coronally advanced to completely cover the graft. Finally, the flap was secured in its final position with 6-0 resorbable sutures (Vicryl Ethicon; Johnson & Johnson Medical, New Brunswick, NJ, USA) (Fig 24). The temporary crown was shortened to avoid any apical pressure on the soft tissues and recemented on the abutment (Fig 25). The same postoperative instructions and medication were provided as after the first surgery.

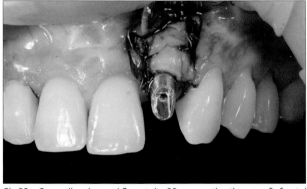

Fig 22   Coronally advanced flap at site 22: connective-tissue graft, frontal view.

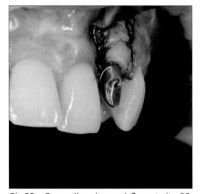

Fig 23   Coronally advanced flap at site 22: connective-tissue graft. profile view.

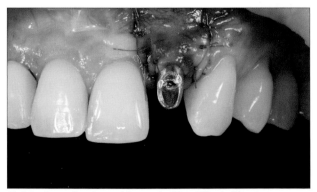

Fig 24   Coronally advanced flap at site 22 stabilized with sutures.

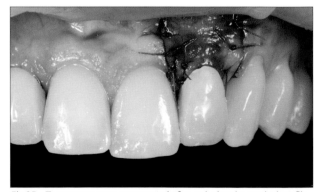

Fig 25   Temporary crown recemented after reducing the cervical profile.

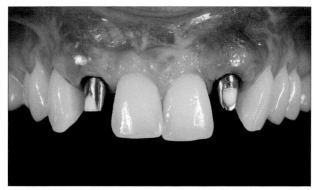

Fig 26 Soft-tissue healing six months after periodontal plastic surgery: frontal view.

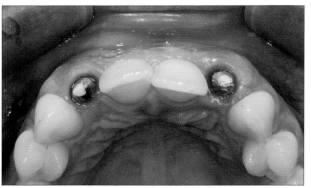

Fig 27 Soft-tissue healing six months after periodontal plastic surgery. occlusal view. Thick and healthy peri-implant soft tissues.

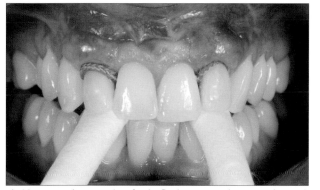

Fig 28 Impression procedure for the final reconstruction: retraction cords gently pushed by the temporary crowns.

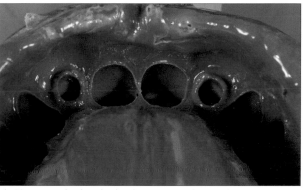

Fig 29 Impression in polyether (Impregum and Permadyne).

Impressions for the final reconstruction

After six months of healing, the peri-implant tissues appeared fully healed and it was possible to confirm the presence of a thick and stable layer of soft tissue around the implants (Figs 26 and 27).

The screw access holes of the abutments were sealed with white composite, and closed-tray impressions for new ceramic crowns were taken using a polyether material (Impregum and Permadyne; 3M Espe, Seefeld, Germany). Prior to impression-taking, the soft tissues were gently retracted with cords placed in the peri-implant sulcus, using the temporary crown to aid insertion (Figs 28 and 29).

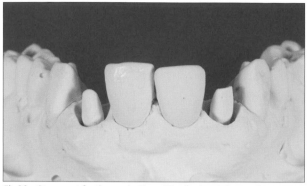

Fig 30   Stone cast for the production of the final metal-ceramic crowns.

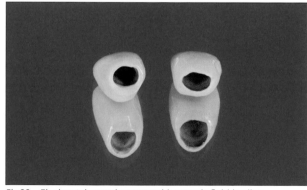

Fig 31   Final metal-ceramic crowns on the stone cast.

Delivery of the final reconstruction

A working model was poured and metal-ceramic crowns were manufactured. To optimize the esthetic result, the dental technician provided a ceramic finishing line (Figs 30 to 32).

After verifying the correct fit and esthetic integration and following approval by the patient, the ceramic crowns were cemented with a glass-ionomer cement (Rely-X Luting, 3M Espe), with the excess cement being carefully removed (Figs 33 to 36).

The final view of the restorations demonstrated a favorable esthetic integration of the crowns in the surrounding soft tissues, and in the smile of the patient. Post cementation radiographs confirmed stability of the peri-implant bone levels and absence of residual cement. The patient declared herself fully satisfied with the outcome of the treatment.

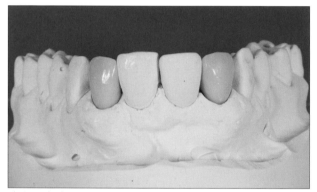

Fig 32   Final metal-ceramic crowns with ceramic finishing line.

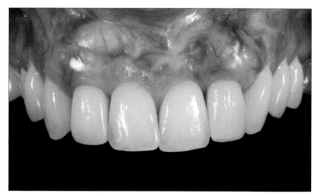

Fig 33   Frontal view of the anterior maxillary teeth after the delivery of the metal-ceramic crowns.

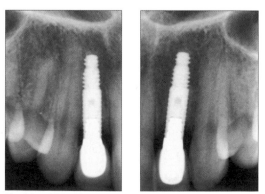

Figs 34 and 35   Final control radiographs.

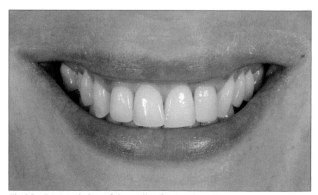

Fig 36   Extraoral view of the smile after treatment.

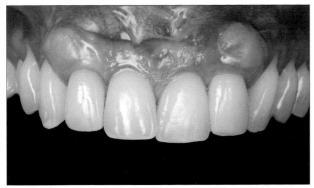

Fig 37   Smile at three years, frontal view.

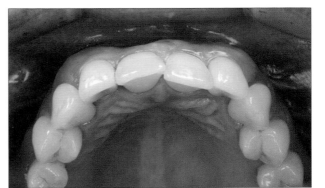

Fig 38   Smile at three years, occlusal view.

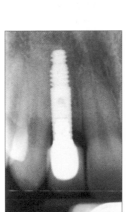

Fig 39   Control radiograph of site 12 at three years.

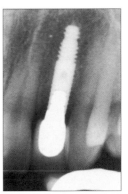

Fig 40   Control radiograph of site 22 at three years.

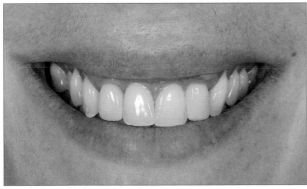

Fig 41   Extraoral view of the smile at three years.

Three-year follow-up

At the three-year clinical and radiological follow-up, the peri-implant soft tissue and bone contours were seen to be stable, with the favorable esthetic outcome being maintained. The patient was recalled every six months for professional oral hygiene and a clinical check-up and has always demonstrated a high standard of oral hygiene. No increased periodontal probing depth and bleeding on probing were recorded at the implant sites at any of the follow-up visits. The control radiographs showed a stable peri-implant bone level. The patient confirmed that her esthetic expectations had been fully met (Figs 37 to 42).

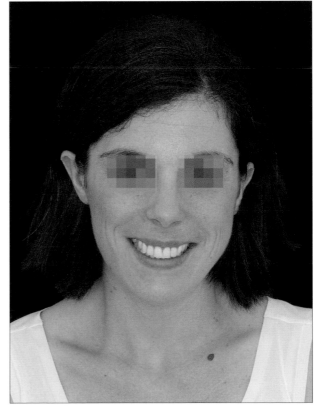

Fig 42   Full-face view at three years.

Discussion

Periodontal plastic surgery to treat soft-tissue dehiscences around dental implants is a relatively recent topic in implant dentistry. Despite limited scientific evidence, mostly comprising case reports and case series, some prospective studies have been published (Burkhardt and coworkers 2008; Zucchelli and coworkers 2013b, 2018b; Roccuzzo and coworkers 2014b) and more recently a literature review (Mazzotti and coworkers 2018). A combined surgical and prosthetic approach (Zucchelli and coworkers 2013b) seems to provide the best results in terms of soft-tissue dehiscence coverage when compared to a pure surgical approach (Burkhardt and coworkers 2018; Roccuzzo and coworkers 2014b).

For this reason, the first treatment step in the present case was aimed at changing the shape of the original implant abutments to provide more space for soft-tissue spontaneous thickening and for the subsequent grafting procedure. Different surgical techniques were utilized for each side. At site 12, the position of the soft-tissue margin was considered adequate, and the treatment goal was mainly soft-tissue thickening to avoid abutment visibility through the soft tissues. A tunnel technique was selected as less invasive (Zuhr and coworkers 2018).

At site 22, the desired treatment outcome was not only soft-tissue thickening but also coronal advancement of the soft-tissue margins through a coronally advanced flap. On both sides, the preferred grafting material was autologous connective tissue, which has demonstrated the best results (Anderson and coworkers 2014 (Burkhardt and coworkers 2008; Zucchelli and coworkers 2013b; Roccuzzo and coworkers 2014b) and it appears to provide satisfactory long-term results (Zucchelli and coworkers 2018b).

Acknowledgments

Laboratory procedures
Alwin Schoenenberger, Vision-Dental – Chiasso, Switzerland and Busto Arsizio, Italy

6.3 GBR and Soft-Tissue Augmentation Following Explantation to Rehabilitate a Soft- and Hard-Tissue Defect

R. Cavalcanti, P. Venezia

Dental implants have become more widespread in recent years—unfortunately sometimes excessively so. A particular problem seems to be that implants are sometimes performed by surgeons who have not enjoyed the benefits of rigorous relevant training.

Dental implants are a valuable resource when resolving situations related to tooth agenesis or loss of teeth due to trauma or illness. They allow esthetics and function to be restored in partially or fully edentulous patients. However, with the increasing number of implants placed, emerging evidence indicates that implants can, over time, lead to a series of technical and, more seriously, biological complications (Derks and coworkers 2016). This presents new challenges in terms of the prevention and treatment of these complications to obtain predictable and stable results over time.

These complications, which must now be considered common, (Giannobile and Lang 2016), often involve not only hard tissues, but also peri-implant soft tissues and can compromise the longevity of implants, with the result that it is sometimes necessary to remove and replace compromised implants.

There have been various proposals for the treatment of peri-implant biological complications so as to preserve the compromised implants, for the treatment of bone defects (Schwartz and coworkers 2012; Roccuzzo and coworkers 2011) and for soft-tissue deficiencies (Burkhardt and coworkers 2008; Zucchelli and coworkers 2013b; Roccuzzo and coworkers 2014b). However, there are no universally accepted protocols for the different complications encountered in the clinical setting. There is even less evidence regarding the protocols to be followed when removing implants and replacing them with new ones.

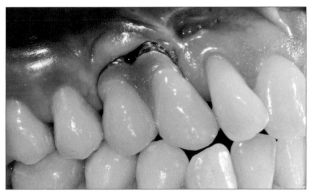

Fig 1   Clinical baseline situation.

The criteria that define an implant as non-salvageable and requiring explantation can include:

- Lack of response to conventional conservative and surgical treatment
- Interference with normal function
- Hazards to the health and stability of the tissues of adjacent teeth or implants
- Implant retention that would imperil the possibility of eventual replacement due to progressive bone destruction

Presenting complaint
A 35-year-old woman, healthy and in good physical condition, presented with esthetic concerns related to an implant-supported restoration replacing teeth 14 and 13 (Fig 1).

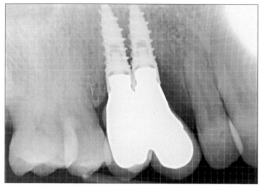

Fig 2   Baseline periapical radiograph. Peri-implant bone loss and proximity of the two implants.

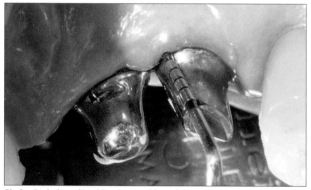

Fig 3   Periodontal/peri-implant probing of the two implants on the palatal aspect.

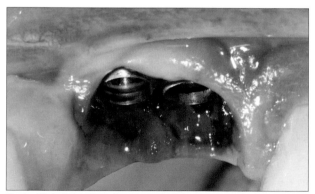

Fig 4   Clinical situation after removal of the crowns and abutments. Inflamed peri-implant mucosa.

Diagnostic aspects and preoperative examination

The patient presented with clinical attachment loss on the proximal and lingual surfaces of the natural dentition. Some gingival recession was present on natural teeth, particularly in the posterior sextants (S1, S3, S4, and S6). Several conservative and prosthetic restorations, some of which would have to be replaced, were also present. At baseline, the full-mouth bleeding score (FMBS) was 54%, while the full-mouth plaque score (FMPS) was 62%, 72% of sites presented with a periodontal probing depth (PPD) of less than 4 mm; 23 % of sites, of 4 to 6 mm; and 5% of sites, of more than 6 mm.

Sextant S1 contained an implant-supported restoration at site 13 – 14, with a large buccal recession defect partially compensated for with pink ceramics applied on the prosthetic device. Teeth 17 and 18 were missing, having been extracted in the past due to caries.

The patient reported that both the implants and the prosthesis had been placed approximately four years previously. The radiographic examination showed significant bone loss around the two implants, particularly in the severely limited interimplant space (Fig 2). Peri-implant probing revealed bleeding on probing (BOP) and 9 mm of pocket depth between the two implants (Fig 3). Tooth 12 was buccally inclined, with gingival recession of about 4 mm, Miller class III (Miller 1985) and Cairo RT2 (Cairo and coworkers 2011). The patient's tissue phenotype was markedly thin (Figs 1 and 4).

The diagnosis was peri-implantitis at implants 13 and 14, with extensive bone loss and extensive buccal mucosal recession as a consequence of incorrect three-dimensional positioning of the implants, which were judged to be untreatable, having been placed in close proximity and preventing appropriate oral hygiene.

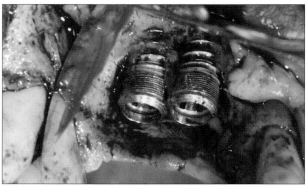

Fig 5   Implants after flap elevation.

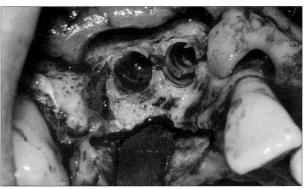

Fig 6   Major residual bone defect after implant removal.

Treatment objectives

The aim was to resolve the functional and esthetic problems in sextants S1 and S2. The following treatment options were considered:

Option 1

Removal of compromised implants; reconstruction of hard and soft tissues; placement of a new standard-diameter implant 14 to support a new prosthesis with a mesial cantilever restoration (Aglietta and coworkers 2009, 2012), and root coverage of 12 by means of periodontal plastic surgery. Using a cantilever extension to replace tooth 13 was suggested because the patient presented with an open bite between teeth 13 and 43 and the lateral guidance was part of the group function on the premolars and first molar.

Option 2

Removal of compromised implants; reconstruction, in a staged approach, of hard and soft tissues: placement of two narrow-diameter implants 14 and 13 with two new implant-supported crowns: root coverage of tooth 12 by means of periodontal plastic surgery.

A further option for the replacement of the missing teeth using a tooth-supported fixed partial denture was rejected due to the length and non-linear shape of the required bridge that would be needed and the additional need for endodontic treatment of the mesial abutment (tooth 12) due to its buccal position and angulation.

It was decided to proceed with Option 1 in order to place as few implants as possible to avoid potential problems arising from interimplant crowding and a lack of access for oral hygiene.

Treatment procedures

An initial phase of non-surgical periodontal therapy, with oral hygiene instructions and motivation using an effective but non-traumatic brushing technique, was followed by a first surgical phase that involved the removal of the compromised implants.

A full-thickness flap was raised to provide adequate access to the implants and surrounding tissues (Fig 5). The implants were removed, leaving a wide through-and-through buccopalatal bone defect with a large vertical component (Fig 6). The need for primary wound closure dictated the use of a free gingival graft to bridge the gap between the buccal and palatal soft tissues. The graft was partially de-epithelialized and placed as an inlay, leaving the epithelialized component exposed (Figs 7 to 12).

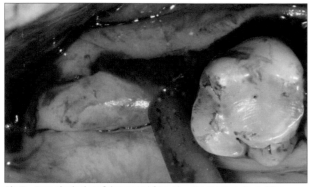

Fig 7   Free gingival graft harvested from the distal edentulous ridge.

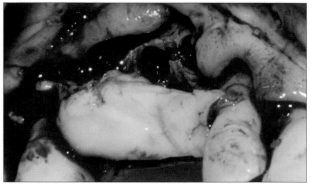

Fig 8   Free gingival graft bridging the gap between the buccal and palatal soft tissues.

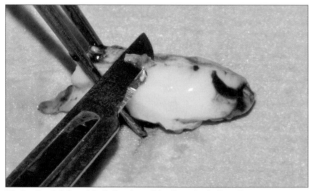

Fig 9   Partial de-epithelialization of the free gingival graft.

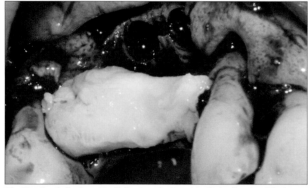

Fig 10   Partially de-epithelialized graft placed in "inlay" style with the epithelized component exposed.

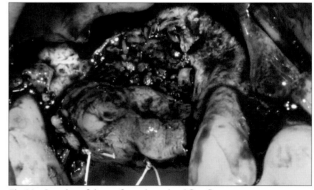

Fig 11   Suturing of the graft, to the palatal flap first, to create a more stable surface on which to anchor the coronally advanced buccal flap.

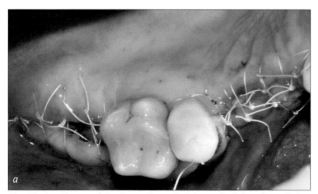

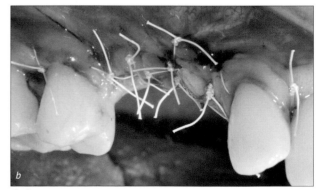

Figs 12a-b   Closure of the donor site and of the grafted site after soft-tissue graft placement.

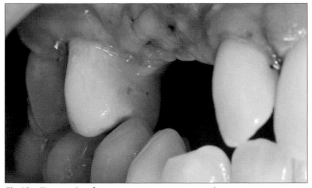

Fig 13   Two weeks after surgery, at suture removal.

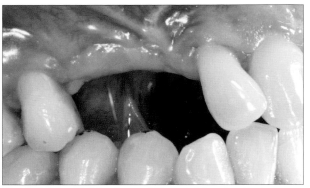

Fig 14   Four months later. Some soft-tissue shrinkage is evident.

The sutures were removed after two weeks (Fig 13) and the patient was recalled every four weeks for the next four months.

Four months later, the patient underwent a second surgery to rebuild the bone tissue lost as a result of peri-implant disease (Figs 14 and 15). Hard-tissue reconstruction was performed by placing small blocks of cortical bone, taken from the mandibular ramus, to create the walls of a box to be filled with autologous bone chips (Figs 16 to 19). A slow-resorbing xenograft layer (DBBM, Bio-Oss; Geistlich Pharma, Wolhusen, Switzerland) was placed on the surface and covered with a resorbable collagen membrane (Bio-Gide; Geistlich Pharma) (Figs 20 and 21). Primary tension-free closure was achieved by the coronal elevation/advancement of the full-thickness flap with periosteal releasing incisions at the bottom/base of the flap while aiming to cover the root of tooth 12 (Fig 22).

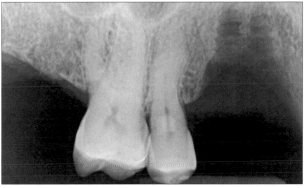

Fig 15   Radiograph of the residual bone defect.

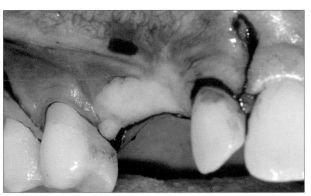

Fig 16   Flap design as part of the second surgical step.

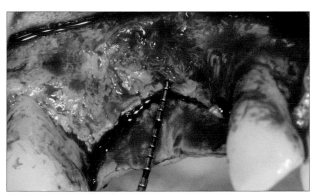

Fig 17   Residual bone defect after flap elevation.

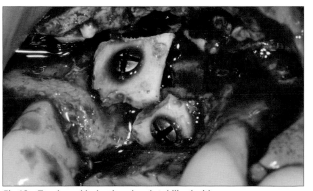

Fig 18   Two bone blocks placed and stabilized with screws.

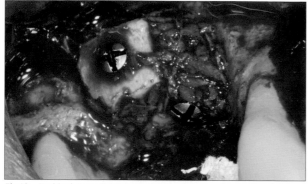

Fig 19 Residual space between the blocks that were filled with autologous bone chips.

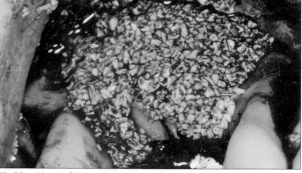

Fig 20 A layer of deproteinized bovine bone placed cover the regenerated site.

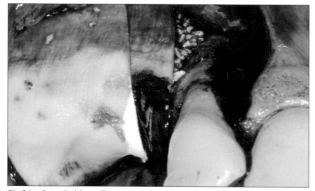

Fig 21 Resorbable collagen membrane placed over the bone graft according to GBR principles.

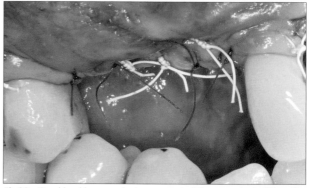

Fig 22 Considerable coronal advancement of the mucogingival line after suturing.

The sutures were removed two weeks later (Figs 23 and 24) and the patient was followed for the next six months.

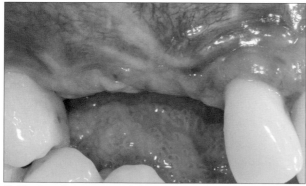

Fig 23 Buccal aspect two weeks later, at suture removal.

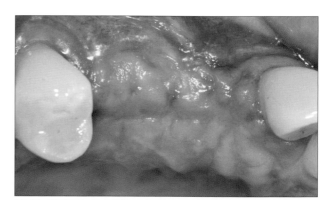

Fig 24 Occlusal view of the wound two weeks after surgery.

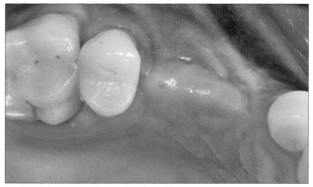
Fig 25   Edentulous ridge at the time of implant surgery.

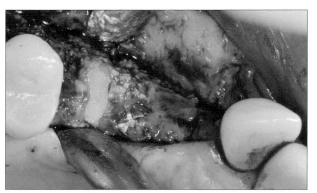
Fig 26   Regenerated bone after flap elevation.

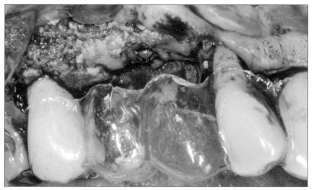
Fig 27   Surgical stent in place.

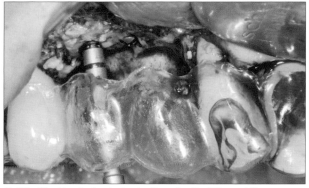
Fig 28   Checking the implant axis after using the 2.2-mm drill.

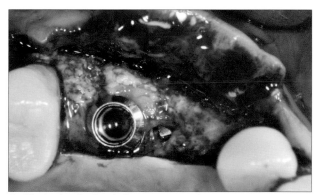
Fig 29   Implant in place before screw removal.

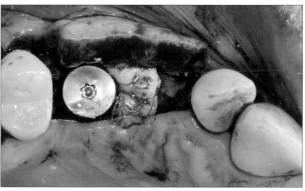
Fig 30   Connective-tissue graft at the mesial aspect of the implant.

At the end of this period, a third operation was performed to insert the planned implants (Figs 25 to 31). As confirmed during the normal preoperative planning phase, it was decided to place only one implant at site 14, replacing tooth 13 with a cantilever extension (Aglietta and coworkers 2009, 2012). An implant (Tissue Level RN Roxolid SLActive, diameter 4.1 mm, length 10 mm; Institut Straumann AG, Basel, Switzerland) was placed simultaneously with a connective-tissue graft mesial to the implant in the pontic region.

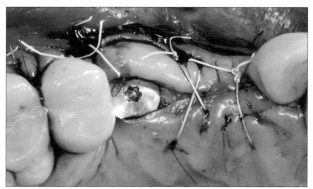
Fig 31   After suturing.

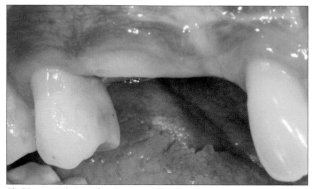

Fig 32   Buccal view after three months of healing.

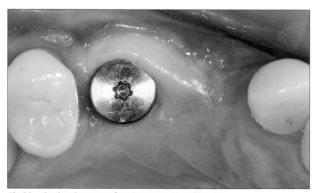

Fig 33   Occlusal aspect after three months of healing.

After a healing period of about three months (Figs 32 and 33), the implant was loaded with a screw-retained provisional restoration with crown 13 attached as a cantilever.

However, edentulous ridge of the canine site had a residual concavity that was corrected by further surgery, placing a connective-tissue graft associated with vestibuloplasty (Figs 34 to 37).

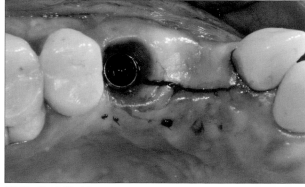

Fig 34   Crestal incision.

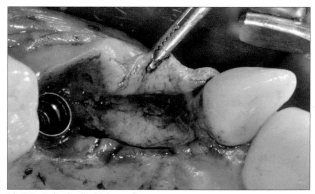

Fig 35   Raised split-thickness flap.

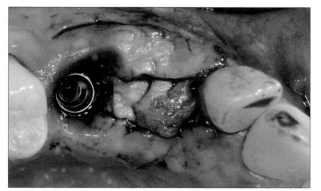

Fig 36   Connective-tissue graft inflating up the edentulous site.

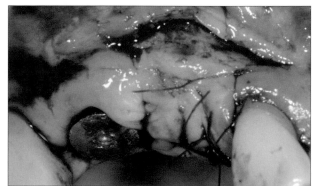

Fig 37   Buccal incision for vestibuloplasty and apical repositioning of the mucogingival line.

Soft-tissue healing and conditioning was guided by means of the temporary restoration; it is ideally suited to this purpose, being relatively simple to modify at chairside by adding or reducing material to exert pressure until satisfactory soft-tissue scalloping has been achieved (Figs 38 to 40).

Once the desired result is obtained, it is important to replicate the soft-tissue profile in the master cast used for the fabrication of the final prosthesis.

Conventional impression techniques are not effective in reproducing the soft-tissue profile because the soft tissues tend to collapse immediately after the removal of the provisional restoration. This is because the soft tissues have been conditioned and individualized during the provisional phase; in many esthetic cases, the transmucosal depth will be deep and difficult to register with a conventional impression.

Since the provisional should perform as an exact replica of the final restoration, it was crucial to transfer the soft-tissue conditioning outcome using a simple, fast, and accurate technique (Hinds 1997) (Fig 41).

First, the provisional restoration was connected to an implant analog and embedded in silicone up to the maximum circumference of the provisional bridge.

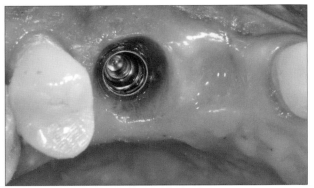

Fig 38   Occlusal view after soft-tissue conditioning.

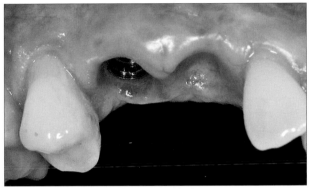

Fig 39   Buccal view after soft-tissue conditioning.

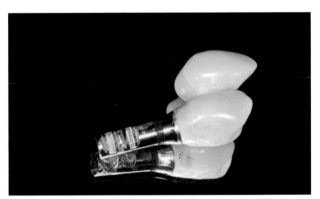

Fig 40   Provisional restoration after progressive chairside modifications.

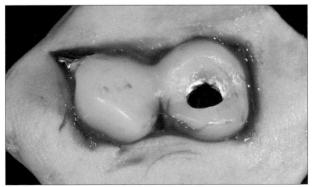

Fig 41   Provisional restoration embedded in silicone for contour registration.

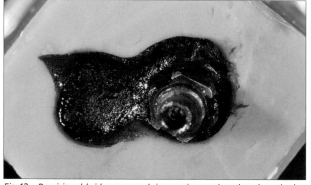

Fig 42 *Provisional bridge removed, impression coping placed on the implant, gap filled with pattern resin.*

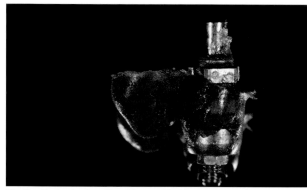

Fig 43 *Customized profile of the modified impression coping.*

As soon as the silicone had set, the provisional restoration was removed and an impression transfer connected to the implant analog. The gap between the impression transfer and the silicone walls of the block was filled with low-shrinkage acrylic resin (Pattern Resin; GC, Tokyo, Japan) (Fig 42).

The customized impression coping (Figs 43 and 44) will allow an accurate transfer of the emergence profile and the pontic area.

The remaining clinical stages are the same as in the standard impression technique (Fig 45). More recently, new techniques have been described for a fully digital approach for the registration of the peri-implant mucosa and pontic areas (Monaco and coworkers 2016; Venezia and coworkers 2017).

The definitive restoration was placed four months later (Figs 46 and 47). It had been planned as a screw-retained monolithic zirconia framework (produced with a milling machine) with feldspathic ceramic veneering limited to the buccal surface (Venezia and coworkers 2015).

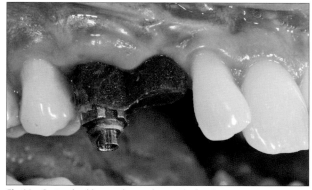

Fig 44 *Customized impression coping on the implant.*

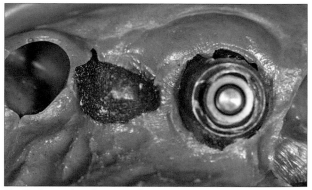

Fig 45 *Impression after removal.*

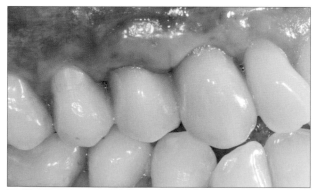

Fig 46 *Final restoration in place.*

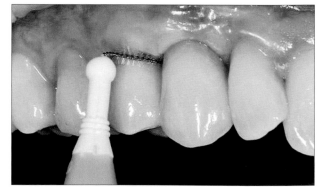

Fig 47 *Good access for oral hygiene.*

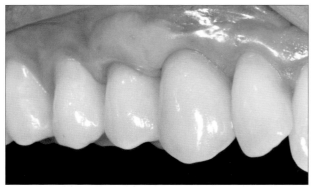

Fig 48   Clinical situation at one year after insertion of the final restoration.

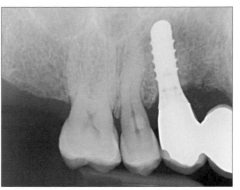

Fig 49   Radiograph, eighteen months later.

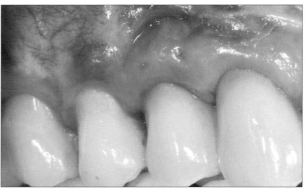

Fig 50   Clinical situation at two years.

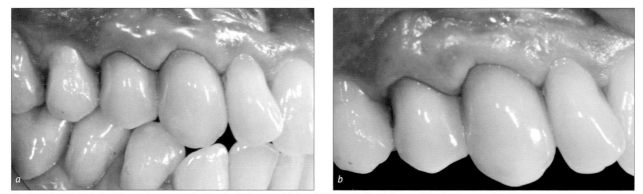

Figs 51a-b   Clinical situation at five years after implant placement (a) and 4.5 years after delivery of the final restoration (b).

At the end of treatment, FMPS was 13% and FMBS was 11%. There was no site with PPD greater than 6 mm, and 14% of sites exhibited a PPD of 4 to 6 mm. The patient was placed on a maintenance program with recall intervals every four months. The patient was greatly satisfied with the result, which was found to be stable at the two-, three- and five-year follow-up visits (Figs 48 to 51).

Discussion

Implants allow us to solve different problems related to edentulism and provide our patients with adequate function and esthetics. However, implants will not infrequently develop various complications of their own, especially in the presence of incorrectly managed risk factors or as the result of incorrect three-dimensional positioning, whether of single implants and of adjacent multiple implants. In particular, placing implants with an excessive buccal angulation in patients with a thin gingival phenotype or inadequate keratinized tissue, may increase the risk of mucosal recession, with consequent exposure of the implant surface. In the case of adjacent implants, failure to provide the proper interimplant distance can increase the risk of "attachment" loss at the interproximal site, creating peri-implant bone defects.

The prevention of such complications is aided by ensuring the stability of the peri-implant tissues through the control of risk factors, in particular smoking, and the absence of residual pockets at the end of periodontal treatment; through correct positioning of the implants the mesiodistal, buccolingual, and apicocoronal directions; through an appropriate choice of implant numbers and implant types; by ensuring minimum interimplant distances; and finally, through proper soft-tissue management, with augmentation performed as needed for functional and esthetic reasons.

In the presence of peri-implant complications, such as bone defects due to peri-implant disease or mucosal recessions on the buccal aspect, various approaches for the treatment and maintenance of compromised implants have been described (Schwartz 2012; Roccuzzo 2011 and 2014b; Zucchelli 2013b; Lang 2001). In case of defects caused by peri-implantitis, treatment proposals vary, ranging from non-surgical and topical pharmacological treatment (Heitz-Mayfield and coworkers 2004; Lang and coworkers 2000), to surgical treatments of a regenerative, resective, or combined nature, with or without implantoplasty. Furthermore, different protocols have been proposed regarding the methods for decontamination of the implant surface.

There is no agreed clinical protocol to determine the need for removing failing implants. A variety of possible clinical situations gives rise to treatment decisions based on individual experience and skill; the available literature consists mainly of case reports, often of purely anecdotal value.

The case presented here is one example of such a clinical situation, with each situation requiring a different approach on a case-by-case basis in terms of both the techniques used and of the surgical sequence. In particular, also as evidenced in the presented case, the correction of peri-implant disease outcomes and the loss of implants frequently require longer treatment times and include many additional steps in order to reach an optimal therapeutic result. Required strategic choices include the number and type of new rehabilitation options aimed at preserving the largest possible volume of reconstructed tissue.

Finally, this case is a clear example of how the reconstruction of soft tissues is often unavoidable to achieve the therapeutic goal and must be performed before or simultaneously with the bone regeneration phase.

Clinical relevance

The decision-making criteria that guide the removal of compromised implants and the protocols to be followed for replacing them with new ones are still difficult to define. However, in case of implant failure, the impact of pathological processes often involves extensive loss of both hard and soft tissues. If the therapeutic choice is to place new implants, the need to rebuild lost (soft and hard) tissues must provide a sequence that, through the reconstruction of soft tissues, improves the healing of the hard tissues and assures their stability in the medium and long term.

Surgical techniques must be used that produce predictable results while reducing, wherever possible, the number of surgical steps and trying to deal with the defects present on adjacent teeth.

6.4 Soft-Tissue Volume Augmentation Using a Connective-Tissue Graft Harvested from the Maxillary Tuberosity

D. Etienne

In 1983, a 51-year-old non-smoking patient was referred for the treatment of moderate chronic periodontitis. At the initial examination, 47% of sites exhibited probing depths of 4 to 6 mm. Periodontal therapy consisted of initial periodontal treatment including oral-hygiene instructions and supra- and subgingival debridement, followed by periodontal surgery to eliminate residual pockets.

Three years following active periodontal therapy, only 8% of sites exhibited residual probing depths of 4 mm, while full-mouth plaque and bleeding scores amounted to 18% and 35%, respectively.

The patient was enrolled in a periodontal maintenance program encompassing regular recall visits every six months, consisting of oral-hygiene instructions, supragingival tooth cleaning, and localized subgingival debridement if needed. The patient also tested positive for a genetic polymorphism of the IL-1 genes (Medical Science System) (Kornman and coworkers 1997).

During the following years, the patient developed endodontic complications, including pulpal necrosis of anterior teeth, which were restored with acid-etched metal/composite-bonded retainers and dentine pins. Vertical root fractures occurred at teeth 36, 37, and 46 (Fig 1), which were subsequently extracted. Tooth 46 was extracted in January 2001 with root separation. The extraction revealed the presence of a deep bony defect on the buccal aspect of the mesial root and a shallow bone defect on the lingual aspect, while the interradicular bone was preserved.

Localized periodontal disease also recurred at teeth 32, 33, and 27, resulting in the loss of tooth 27.

In March 2001, the patient was treated for a myocardial infarction that involved the placement of a stent. The cardiologist's approval to proceed with implant placement was received in November 2002 (the patient was 70 years old at that time) (Fig 2).

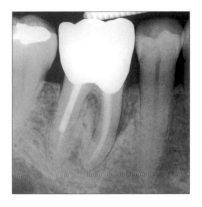

Fig 1 During a scheduled periodontal-maintenance visit, a vertical root fracture of the mesial root of tooth 46 was diagnosed. The intraoperative radiograph revealed the presence of an intrabony defect at the mesial surface of the mesial root.

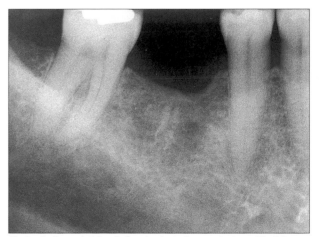

Fig 2 Radiograph taken before implant placement at age 70, 1.5 years after a myocardial infarction.

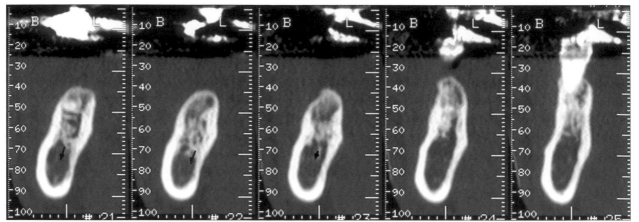

Fig 3   Limited crestal resorption buccally on the mesial aspect of the edentulous ridge.

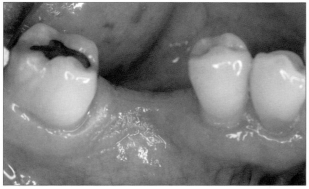

Fig 4   Buccal view two years after extraction indicated a slight horizontal volume deficiency.

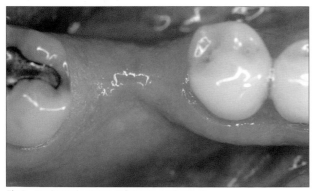

Fig 5   Horizontal volume deficiency, occlusal view.

The sagittal scan revealed limited crestal resorption buccally on the mesial aspect of the edentulous ridge (Fig 3).

The clinical situation two years after the extraction of tooth 46 demonstrated the presence of an adequate width of keratinized mucosa, with the mucogingival line in the edentulous space located slightly coronally to that of the adjacent teeth. The alveolar ridge appeared to have a slight horizontal volume deficiency (Figs 4 and 5).

Despite the horizontal volume deficiency, the bone volume and the soft-tissue characteristics appeared to favor single-stage implant placement in conjunction with immediate soft-tissue augmentation to compensate for the missing buccal soft-tissue concavity by means of a dense connective-tissue graft, harvested from the tuberosity, to eliminate the need for a more invasive bone-regeneration procedure. At the same time, this approach would reduce the surgical trauma by limiting the number of procedures to a single one, minimizing the healing time needed for the prosthetic reconstruction.

Soft-tissue augmentation using a connective-tissue graft harvested from the palate or tuberosity has been used to compensate for ridge defects prior to conventional bridge rehabilitations, where outcomes remained stable for up to 10 years (Seibert and Salama 1996). An obvious

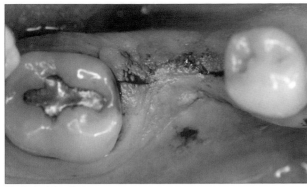

Fig 6   Incision design.

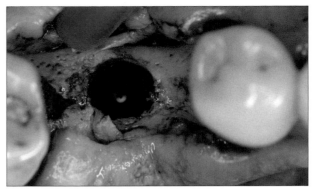

Fig 7   Prepared implant bed.

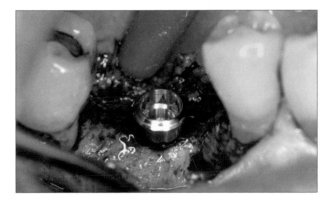

Fig 8   Inserted tissue-level implant, buccal view.

advantage of connective-tissue grafts from the tuberosity is their reduced morbidity. Therefore, if available—and surgically accessible—the area of the tuberosity is an appropriate donor site for the management of both gingival recessions (Azzi and coworkers 1991) and ridge defects.

Additionally, connective-tissue grafts can be used to increase the thickness of the gingival tissue, thus changing the local phenotype (Jung and coworkers 2008), or to increase soft-tissue volume (Sanz-Martín and coworkers 2018).

Following a submerged approach for securing the connective-tissue graft harvested from the tuberosity, the wound healed quickly and without complications, which resulted in a clinically satisfactory gain in buccal volume, observed already after two months. At the donor site, wound healing is rarely delayed, and patients experience limited pain compared to palatal donor sites (Amin and coworkers 2018). A practical advantage of connective-tissue grafts harvested from the tuberosity is related to the clinical handling of the graft, which can be easily trimmed to the configuration of the defect and, if needed, stabilized with submerged periosteal sutures after a releasing incision on the inside of the buccal flap. In comparison, GBR procedures in the posterior mandible, including membrane stabilization, are technically more challenging, and the required healing time will exceed six months. Additionally, a GBR procedure cannot always be performed in one single stage.

Surgical procedure

A crestal incision was made slightly lingually to the anticipated implant position (Fig 6). Full-thickness flaps were elevated, with a limited envelope on the buccal and lingual aspects of the adjacent teeth (Fig 7). Following preparation of the implant site, the remaining buccal bone wall was found to be thin. The crestal bone was evaluated during surgery with Type II bone density during drilling (Lekholm and Zarb 1985), with 1 mm in thickness and Type III medullary bone density.

A tissue-level implant (TE RN SLA, diameter 4.1 mm, length 12 mm; Institut Straumann AG, Basel, Switzerland) was accommodated within the bony envelope (Fig 8).

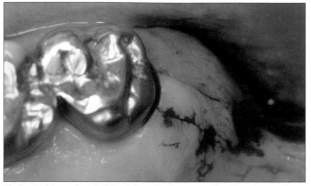

Fig 9   Incisions placed at the tuberosity for connective-tissue harvesting.

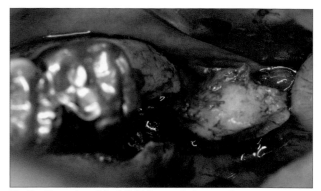

Fig 10   Harvesting of the full-thickness soft-tissue graft.

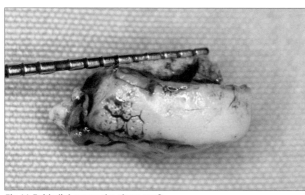

Fig 11 Epithelial connective-tissue graft.

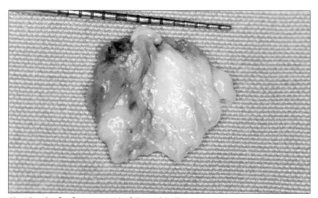

Fig 12   Graft after removal of the epithelium.

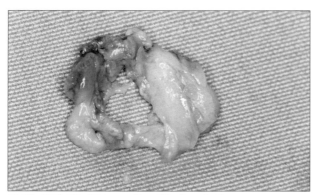

Fig 13   Graft after the preparation of the "poncho."

The left maxillary tuberosity was shallow but offered a more favorable volume than the right side. A palatal incision was made and directed towards the distolingual line angle of the second molar, with a parallel incision placed 3 mm toward the buccal aspect (Fig 9). A deep horizontal releasing incision was placed to connect the two parallel incisions, facilitating the harvesting of the connective-tissue graft.

The buccal and palatal flaps were thinned using internal beveled incisions and reflected to full thickness to allow harvesting of an optimal volume of connective tissue (Schluger and coworkers 1977) (Fig 10). The full-thickness soft-tissue graft obtained was thick, with a sufficient vertical component (Fig 11).

The epithelial layer was removed with a #15 blade; the remaining connective tissue was split vertically. The increased surface of the remaining connective-tissue graft was dense, with an approximate thickness of 1,5 mm (Fig 12).

Since no vertical releasing incision was used at the buccal recipient site, the connective-tissue graft was prepared using a "poncho" technique (Fig 13). Using small incisions, a thin collar of tissue was prepared to passively retain the graft on the lingual aspect of the implant, covering around 2 mm of the healing abutment, while the remaining buccal part of the graft measured around 5 mm in height.

D. Etienne

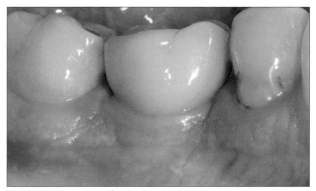

Fig 23 Fourteen years after implant loading.

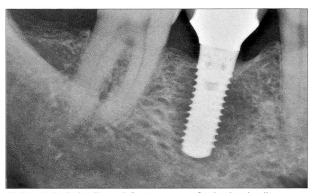

Fig 24 Periapical radiograph fourteen years after implant loading.

The clinical evaluation fourteen years after prosthetic restoration revealed a stable buccal soft-tissue margin and interproximal papillae. The keratinized mucosa width was 3.5 mm on the buccal and 4 mm on the lingual aspect, with probing depths of 4 mm both buccally and lingually. Slight bleeding on probing was noted lingually, with exposed crown measurements of 6 mm on the buccal and lingual aspects (Fig 23).

Over the years, the soft-tissue margin remained stable buccally and even revealed some slight marginal creep coronally. Lingually, however, some slight recession of the soft tissue occurred during the first five years. The probing depth was unchanged over time both buccally and lingually, indicating peri-implant tissue stability. The intraoral radiographs at five and fourteen years revealed no differences, indicating stability of the marginal bone (Fig 24).

Conclusion

The present clinical case illustrates the possibility of using a dense connective-tissue graft of moderate thickness harvested from the tuberosity to compensate for a buccal soft-tissue deficit, despite thin buccal bone. Long-term volume stability with 2 mm of peri-implant bone has been shown in a case series for single implants and connective-tissue grafts from the palate (Hanser and Khoury 2016). A similar potential of connective-tissue grafts from the palate and tuberosity to compensate for soft-tissue defects at single implants has also been reported, but only in a short-term study (Rojo and coworkers 2018).

The stability of peri-implant buccal bone may point to a protective effect of the connective-tissue graft on the cortical buccal plate, probably due to the increase in mucosal thickness (Bengazi and coworkers 2015).

Acknowledgment

Prosthetic procedures
Dr. Richard Joly – Paris, France

6.5 Connective-Tissue Graft to Increase the Width of the Keratinized Mucosa Around an Osseointegrated Implant

V. Iorio-Siciliano

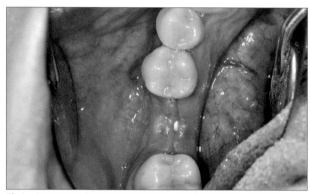

Fig 1   Premature-closure screw exposure with inadequate keratinized mucosa.

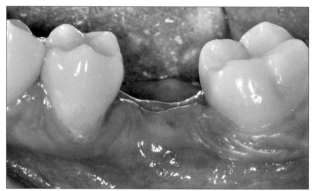

Fig 2   Thin residual keratinized mucosa on the buccal aspect.

A healthy 38-year-old woman, a non-smoker, was referred to Department of Periodontology of the University of Naples in May 2014 for increasing the width of the keratinized tissues at the buccal aspect of dental implant 46. The site exhibited a premature-closure screw exposure caused by trauma during chewing, with inadequate keratinized tissue (Fig 1).

The phenotype of the keratinized mucosa was thin. The patient complained of pain during toothbrushing in the region (Fig 2).

The tooth was lost due to a vertical fracture. Six months following its extraction, an implant had been placed without any additional GBR.

The main objective of the treatment plan was to increase the height and thickness of the peri-implant soft tissues to obtain a stable mucosal seal and a width of keratinized tissue favorable to toothbrushing. It has been suggested that an inadequate height and thickness of the peri-implant keratinized tissue may result in increased plaque accumulation, higher rates of peri-implant mucositis, and a higher risk of soft-tissue dehiscence (Chung and coworkers 2006; Bouri and coworkers 2008; Adibrad and coworkers 2009; Schrott and coworkers 2009; Boynuegri and coworkers 2013).

The recommended treatment plan was to create an access flap in combination with a subepithelial autologous connective-tissue graft for augmenting the buccal site (Thoma and coworkers 2009; Bassetti and coworkers 2016). The rationale of the treatment was discussed, and written consent was obtained. The patient presented with good oral hygiene. Both the full-mouth bleeding score (FMBS) and the full-mouth plaque score (FMPS) were less than 62%, and the full-mouth probing chart did not reveal any pockets with depths of 4 mm or more.

Under local anesthesia, a full-thickness mucoperiosteal flap was elevated extending one tooth width in the mesial and distal direction on the buccal and lingual aspects. The closure screw was removed and replaced with a taller healing abutment 5.0 mm in diameter and 5.0 mm in height. The connective-tissue graft was harvested using the deepithelialized gingival graft technique described by Zucchelli and coworkers (2010). The graft was anchored on the internal aspect of the buccal flap by two internal horizontal mattress sutures using a 5-0 non-resorbable material (Fig 3).

Two interrupted sutures were placed further coronally to adapt the buccal and lingual flaps around the healing abutment (Fig 4).

The palatal donor site was sutured with a sling mattress suture (Vicryl 4-0) to achieve palatal healing by secondary intention. Postoperative pain was controlled with ibuprofen (600 mg immediately before the surgical intervention and after 4 hours). The patient was instructed not to brush her teeth in the treated areas and to rinse with a chlorhexidine solution (0.12%) three times a day for one minute. No systemic antibiotics were prescribed. The sutures were removed one week after surgery. Professional supragingival tooth cleaning with a rubber cup and chlorhexidine gel was performed during the first four weeks after surgery. After this time, the patient was instructed to resume normal oral hygiene and to discontinue the chlorhexidine. After a six-month observation period, excellent soft-tissue integration was observed (Figs 5 and 6) and a provisional acrylic single crown was cemented.

The cemented definitive metal-ceramic single crown was delivered after one month (Fig 7).

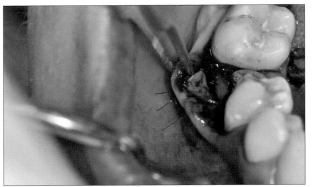

Fig 3   Connective-tissue graft anchored on the internal aspect of the buccal flap.

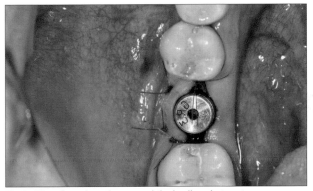

Fig 4   Flap after adaptation around the healing abutment.

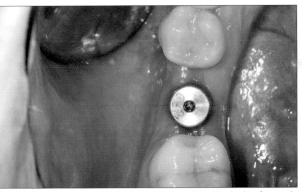

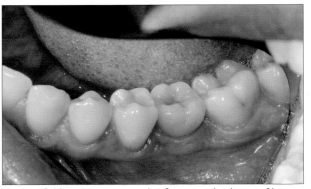

Fig 5   After six months of soft-tissue healing with the gingiva former in place.

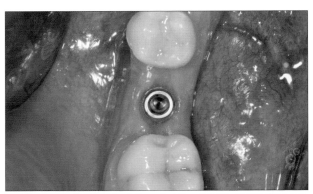

Fig 6   After six months of soft-tissue healing with the gingiva former removed.

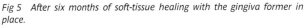

Fig 7   Definitive crown seven months after connective-tissue grafting.

Discussion

Generally, this surgical approach is often proposed for the anterior area to improve the esthetic outcome, with the subepithelial connective-tissue grafting technique providing a simultaneous vertical and horizontal soft-tissue increase around single implants (Stefanini and coworkers 2016).

In the anterior region, in the presence of a thin ridge, implant placement without simultaneous GBR will often be possible but leave a residual concavity in the soft tissues on the buccal aspect. Results from a recent clinical study have shown that this type of peri-implant soft-tissue defect can be corrected with a connective-tissue graft (De Bruvckere and coworkers 2018).

However, increased peri-implant soft-tissue thickness is essential not only for esthetic but also for functional reasons. A recent consensus report found that soft-tissue grafting to increase the width of keratinized tissue around implants is associated with reduced plaque accumulation and less inflammation of the peri-implant mucosa compared to non-augmented sites (Giannobile and coworkers 2018). Although scientific evidence is lacking, soft-tissue augmentation at implant sites should also be considered (Cairo and coworkers 2008) in the posterior area if needed, to promote peri-implant health.

The clinical result obtained in the posterior area in this case is in agreement with outcomes reported in a previous study (Wiesner and coworkers 2010). The authors reported that implants treated with a connective-tissue graft showed a greater thickness of the peri-implant soft tissues (1.3 mm) and were associated with greater patient satisfaction than those who did not undergo this clinical procedure.

The peri-implant soft tissues may play an important role in preventing marginal bone loss (Berglundh and Lindhe 1996). In fact, in the presence of a thin (less than 2 mm) band of peri-implant karatinized attached mucosa (Linkevicius 2009), the development of biologic width may cause crestal bone resorption, while marginal bone loss is significantly reduced if the attached mucosa is thick (2 mm or more) (Suárez-López del Amo and coworkers 2016).

Various approaches to the second-stage surgery (U-shaped or T-shaped incision) have been proposed to increase the thickness of the peri-implant mucosa in the presence of an adequate width of attached mucosa (Grossberg 2001; Shahidi and coworkers 2008). Unfortunately, these techniques were not suitable in the present case, since the amount of keratinized tissue was too limited. The need to significantly increase the amount of attached mucosa meant that there were two surgical options available: a free gingival graft or a coronally repositioned flap in combination with a connective-tissue graft.

The latter approach was chosen to simplify the surgical procedure and to achieve transmucosal wound healing. Usually, this approach is based on a partial-thickness flap, and the connective-tissue graft is anchored to the periosteum to stimulate adequate vascularization (Mazzotti and coworkers 2018). However, in the present case, the residual keratinized mucosa was too thin; elevating a partial-thickness flap would probably have caused flap perforation, resulting in further soft-tissue dehiscence. Therefore, a full-thickness flap was elevated, and the connective-tissue graft was anchored to the buccal flap, which, being a pedicle flap, guaranteed vascularization.

This choice of clinical approach was based on previous results. Speroni and coworkers (2010) placed connective-tissue grafts on the buccal aspect of implants during second-stage surgery, increasing the thickness of the mucosa by an average of 2.14 mm. These outcomes are corroborated by Papapetros and coworkers (2019), who reported an average increase in mucosal thickness of 2.60 ± 1.27 mm for sites treated with an access flap and a connective-tissue graft. Nevertheless, studies with longer follow-up periods are needed to assess the stability of the peri-implant tissues over time.

6.6 Soft- and Hard-Tissue Regeneration and Implant-Supported Restorations to Treat a Complex Anterior Maxillary Case

R. Jung, A. Gil, C. Hämmerle, D. Thoma

A 19-year-old man presented at the clinic with esthetic concerns regarding his maxillary anterior teeth. The patient was a male student, a non-smoker and occasional drinker. His chief complaint was "a retained tooth that is out of position." He reported being very displeased with his esthetic situation.

The patient was an ASA type I patient with a non-contributory medical history and no drug allergies.

At the age of twelve, the patient suffered a traumatic injury in the maxillary anterior region, resulting in the loss of teeth 12 and 11. Tooth 21 suffered a partial luxation and was repositioned in the socket. This tooth became ankylosed, causing a significant vertical discrepancy of the soft-tissue margin and of the incisal edge (Fig 1). The patient underwent orthodontic treatment with a mesial shift of all maxillary right teeth to move tooth 13 to site 12.

Diagnosis and treatment plan

The patient was partially edentulous, with missing teeth 12 and 11. Tooth 13 was at position of 12 with an orthodontic device in place. The periodontal diagnosis was localized plaque-induced gingivitis, with pockets ranging from 2 to 4 mm but without loss of attachment, a full-mouth plaque score of 10%, and a modified sulcular bleeding index of 0.7 ± 0.2. Due to the trauma and the resorption of the ridge, the patient exhibited a Seibert class III ridge at the edentulous site 11. Tooth 21 presented with early ankylosis. The overall prognosis of his teeth was good, with the exception of tooth 21, whose prognosis was poor due to its ankylosed status and severe infraposition.

The treatment plan for this patient consisted of (Fig 2):
- Scaling and root planing and oral hygiene instructions
- Removal of the orthodontic wires and shortening crown 21 (as far subgingivally as possible) to create space for soft-tissue ingrowth in anticipation of an improvement in the soft-tissue situation
- Extraction of tooth 21 with flap elevation and simultaneous soft-tissue augmentation
- Bone augmentation with an autologous block graft and a resorbable membrane
- Placement of two implants 11 and 21
- Delivery of two all-ceramic crowns 11 and 21 and a composite veneer on tooth 13 to mimic tooth 12

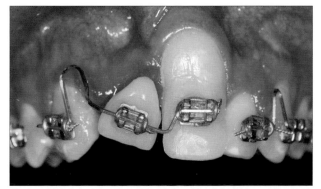

Fig 1   Initial clinical situation with ankylosed tooth 21 with an orthodontic device.

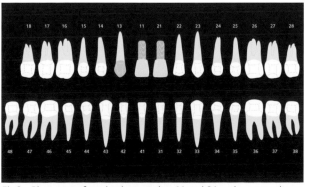

Fig 2   Placement of two implants at sites 11 and 21 and a composite veneer on tooth 13 to mimic tooth 12.

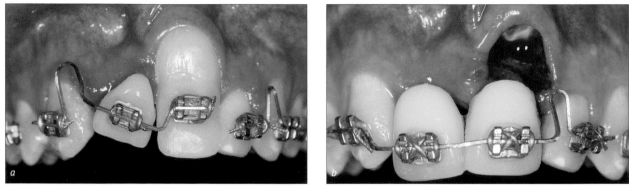

Figs 3a-b   Ankylosed tooth 21 before (a) and after (b) shortening of the crown.

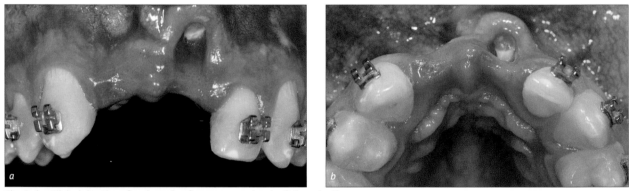

Figs 4a-b   Clinical situation after six weeks of crown removal and soft-tissue healing.

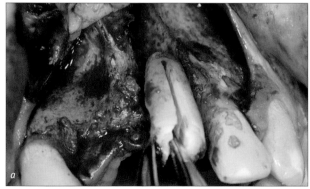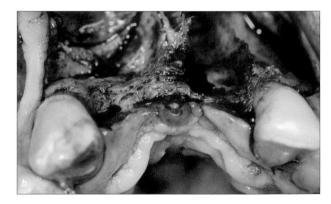

Figs 5a-b   Extraction of tooth 21 with a severe alveolar defect.

Surgical phase

The ankylosis of tooth 21 had placed its gingival margin in a markedly apical position, causing a severe vertical soft- and hard-tissue deficiency and, consequently, an esthetic problem (Fig 3a). Using a diamond bur, the crown of tooth 21 was reduced as close as possible to the bone level (Fig 3b) to allow the soft tissue to heal, improving its quality and quantity before the surgical extraction of the remaining root tip. The situation had improved after six weeks of healing, and the space previously occupied by the crown had substantially closed and healed over the remaining root (Figs 4a-b).

After elevating a full-thickness flap with a releasing incision distal to tooth 22, the remaining root 21 was carefully extracted using a diamond bur and straight elevators. The socket was curetted and irrigated with saline. Due to the soft-tissue margin discrepancy, surgical soft-tissue augmentation was indicated prior to any bone or implant surgery (Figs 5a-b).

A connective-tissue graft was harvested from the palate and stabilized over the defect to improve the quality and quantity of the overlying soft tissue and to allow for future bone augmentation with stable soft-tissue conditions (Figs 6a-c). The postoperative photograph illustrates the healing progress after eight weeks, with increased mucosal thickness and vertical height.

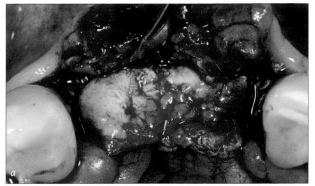

Figs 6a-c   Soft-tissue augmentation with a subepithelial connective-tissue graft harvested from the palate.

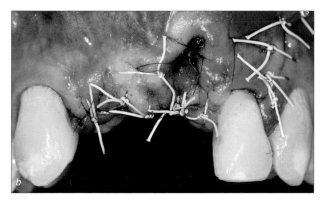

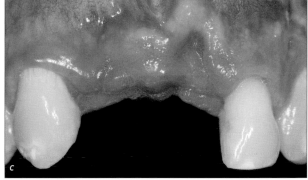

Once the soft tissue had completely healed, a staged bone augmentation procedure was performed. A block graft from the mandibular symphysis was harvested and secured to the recipient site with screws. In addition, a bone mineral substitute (Bio-Oss; Geistlich, Wolhusen, Switzerland), was placed and a resorbable collagen membrane (Bio-Gide; Geistlich) was used to cover both bone grafts, which were left to heal for six months (Figs 7a-c).

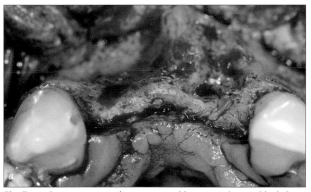

Figs 7a-c   Bone augmentation surgery with an autologous block bone graft, bone substitute material, and a resorbable collagen membrane.

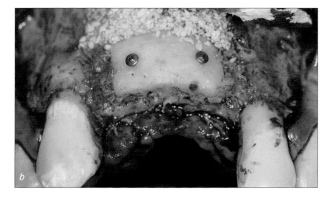

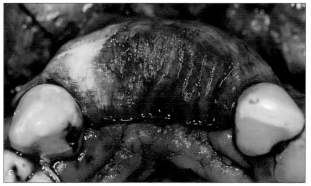

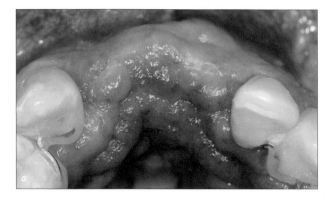

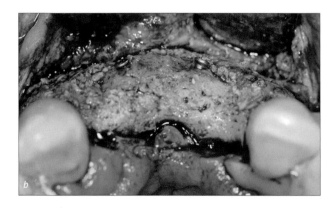

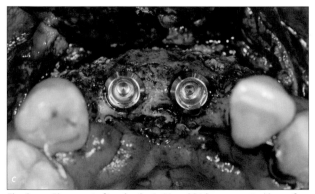

Figs 8a-c   Placement of two implants 11 and 21 in regenerated bone, four months after bone augmentation.

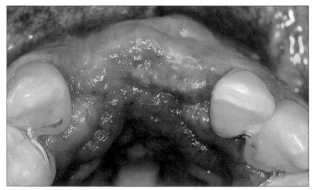

Fig 9   Before abutment connection.

After four months of healing, two implants, 11 and 21, were planned using a restorative-driven approach. A full-thickness flap with one vertical releasing incision was raised, the fixation screws were removed and two implants (Standard Plus, RN, diameter 4.1 mm, length 12 mm; Institut Straumann AG, Basel, Switzerland) were placed with high primary stability in adequate circumferential bone at sites 11 and 21 (Figs 8a-c). Cover screws were then connected and the implants left to heal in a submerged protocol for four months. A removable provisional restoration was provided during the healing period.

Abutment connection surgery was performed four months after implant placement. A minimal access flap was used to remove the cover screws (Figs 9), and two healing abutments were placed.

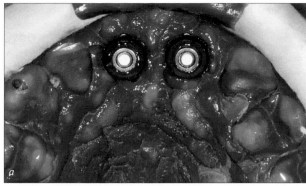
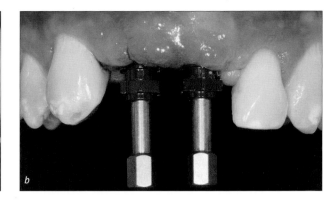

Figs 10a-b   Open-tray impressions of implants 11 and 21.

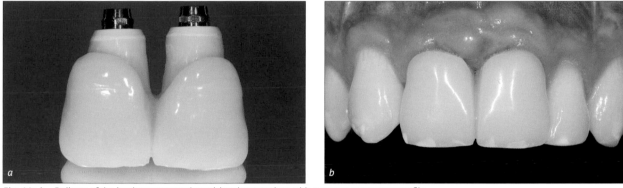

Figs 11a-b   Delivery of the implant-supported provisional restorations with a narrow emergence profile.

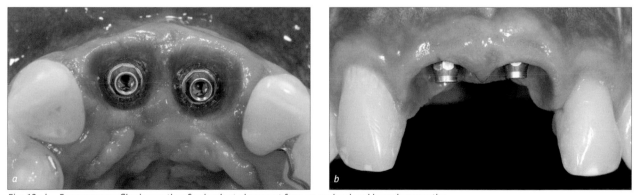

Figs 12a-b   Emergence profile six months after implant placement from an occlusal and buccal perspective.

Prosthetic phase

Six weeks after the abutment connection, open-tray impressions were taken of the implants 11 and 21 (Figs 10a-b). The impressions were sent to the dental laboratory for fabrication of splinted screw-retained provisional restorations, which were delivered eight weeks after abutment-connection surgery to shape the soft-tissue emergence profile (Figs 11a-b).

During the first four to six weeks, the emergence profile of the provisional restoration was modified by selectively adding flowable composite (Tetric Flow; Ivoclar Vivadent, Schaan, Liechtenstein) to mimic the natural appearance of a tooth. In addition, the soft tissue was superficially shaped with a diamond bur to reduce the irregularities and scar tissue of the peri-implant mucosa. The patient wore the provisional restorations for another four months to allow soft-tissue maturation (Figs 12a-b). For the definitive prosthetic reconstruction, two In-Ceram abutments (Institut Straumann AG) were directly veneered with feldspathic ceramic.

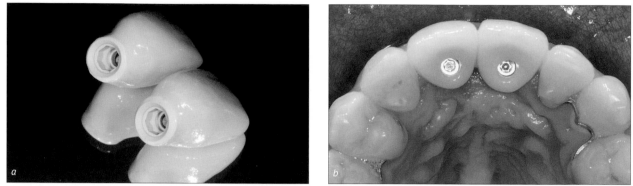

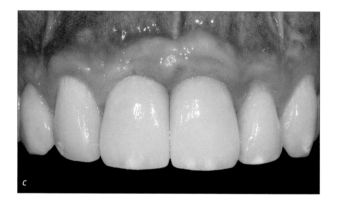

Figure 13a-c   Clinical situation two years after the delivery of the implant crowns.

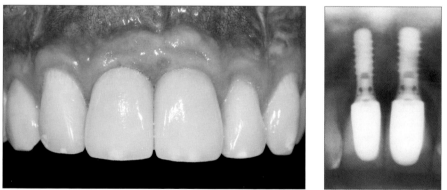

Fig 14   Two years after restoration delivery.

Fig 15   Periapical radiograph at the two-year follow-up, with stable marginal bone levels.

At the time of the delivery of crowns 11 and 21, a direct composite restoration was also built up on tooth 13 (at site 12), mimicking a lateral incisor. The implant-supported all-ceramic crowns were screw-retained using 35 Ncm of torque, and the access holes were filled with PTFE tape and a composite filling material. The patient was satisfied with their fit and esthetic appearance (Figs 13a-c).

No complications occurred during the follow-up period. The situation at two years shows stable clinical results (full-mouth plaque score of 8% and a modified sulcular bleeding index of 0.5 ± 0.1), with healthy peri-implant soft tissue and an esthetically pleasing reconstruction (Fig 14). The two-year follow-up radiograph also shows stable marginal bone levels (Fig 15).

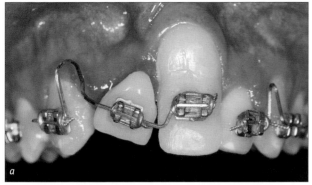

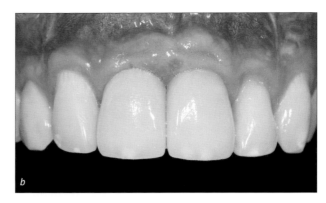

Figs 16a-b   Comparison of the pre- and postoperative situation.

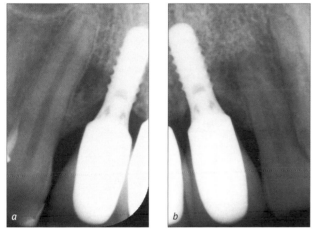

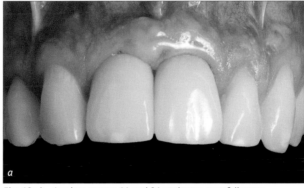

Figs 18a-b   Implant crowns 11 and 21 at the ten-year follow-up.

Figs 17a-b   Periapical radiographs of implants 11 and 21 at the ten-year follow-up.

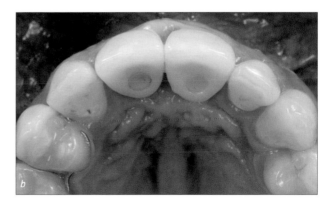

The patient's chief complaint was addressed by creating a healthy situation and providing him with esthetically pleasing reconstructions. The definitive implant crowns were screw-retained and all-ceramic. The symmetry of the gingival margin and incisal edges was restored. The patient was very satisfied with the result after two years (Figs 16a-b).

The patient was recently recalled for a ten-year follow-up. The radiographs (Figs 17a-b) indicated stable marginal bone levels, while the clinical examination revealed healthy peri-implant mucosa with functional implant crowns (Figs 18a-b).

Discussion

The presented complex maxillary anterior case involved comprehensive treatment, considering diagnosis, soft- and hard-tissue management, implant surgery, and prosthetic rehabilitation. It illustrates the importance of orchestrating all treatment steps in a meticulous and multidisciplinary approach. It also emphasizes that a stable long-term result can be achieved when each individual treatment step is successfully completed.

Soft-tissue augmentation. The initial clinical presentation did not allow any bone or implant surgery to be performed without first improving the soft-tissue situation. Soft-tissue augmentation was therefore mandated. There was a significant discrepancy between the gingival margins of the two central incisors and a concomitant lack of keratinized mucosa and deficient volume in this area.

A severe apical position of the gingival margin around an ankylosed tooth implies a greater risk of developing peri-implant mucosal recession if left untreated. From an esthetic point of view, the gray color of the titanium implant and the implant components may cause major problems when exposed due to peri-implant mucosal recession (Glauser and coworkers 2014; Kohal and coworkers 2008; Evans and Chen 2008), which can dramatically compromise the esthetic appearance of the restoration (Burkhardt and coworkers 2000; Roccuzzo and coworkers 2014b).

In the presented case, tooth 21 exhibited a narrow band of keratinized mucosa due to the severe apical position of the gingival margin. A lack of keratinized mucosa has been correlated with more plaque accumulation, more mucosal inflammation, a high risk of mucosal recession, and an impaired ability to perform proper maintenance (Gobbato and coworkers 2013; Brito and coworkers 2014; Souza and coworkers 2016). At the outset, a deficient mucosal volume was evident at both future implant sites 11 and 21, which may have a negative impact on the final esthetic result of the implant treatment (Jung and coworkers 2007, 2008a) and may also have a negative effect on peri-implant marginal bone levels (Linkevicius and coworkers 2009; Puisys and Linkevicius 2015; Akcalı and coworkers 2017).

For all the above-mentioned reasons and to provide a thicker mucosa ahead of bone augmentation surgery, soft-tissue augmentation was planned using a subepithelial connective-tissue graft harvested from the palate and secured with sutures on the crestal and buccal sides of the ridge. The choice of this graft material is based on the consideration that an autologous graft is still considered the gold standard for volume augmentation in terms of tissue stability and thickness gain (Cortellini and Pino Prato 2012; Chambrone and Tatakis 2015). There are some soft-tissue substitutes that have shown promising results (Thoma and coworkers 2018a), but long-term data is still lacking.

Bone augmentation. Because of the traumatic injury, the ankylosed condition of tooth 11, and the extended period of partial edentulism, the maxillary anterior ridge was significantly resorbed and did not permit implant placement in an optimal, prosthetically driven position. Adequate bone volume is a prerequisite for implant placement, and the situation required substantial ridge augmentation to increase both the height and the width of the ridge. A plethora of ridge preservation and augmentation procedures have been described for different indications (Benic and Hämmerle 2014), but in the severely resorbed ridge, the use of autologous bone blocks, alone or in combination with bone substitutes or collagen membranes, is the treatment of choice (Jensen and Terheyden 2009; Klein and Al-Nawas 2011). The goal is to achieve a facial thickness of the buccal bone of at least 2 mm, which is thought to maintain adequate marginal bone levels around the implant over time (Spray and coworkers 2000).

Accordingly, a bone augmentation procedure was planned using a combination of an autologous block graft from the mandibular symphysis and a particulate xenograft, covered by a resorbable collagen membrane. The membrane was utilized with a view to decreasing the resorption of the autologous block (Maiorana and coworkers 2005; von Arx and Buser 2006) and to reduce the risk of complications (Jung and coworkers 2009, 2013). It has been suggested that a proper incision design and adequate release of the periosteum are key factors for tension-free wound closure (Tinti and Parma-Benfenati 1998; Simion and coworkers 2007). This was achieved here by a combination of periosteal releasing incisions and the use of horizontal mattress and single interrupted sutures. No complications occurred during the postoperative healing period, so the implant could be placed four months later. Soft-tissue augmentation prior to any bone augmentation procedures might contribute to uneventful healing.

Implant placement. After the bone and soft-tissue management procedures, the situation was stable and the implantation could proceed. Two tissue level implants were planned for sites 11 and 21. The implant position was prosthetically planned to accommodate a screw-retained reconstruction. This was possible because grafted bone was present on the buccal side, allowing the implant to be placed in a prosthetically driven three-dimensional position. From a horizontal perspective, implants were placed 3 mm apart to allow for a greater interproximal tissue fill (Tarnow and coworkers 2000; Ramanauskaite and coworkers 2018). Tissue Level implants were chosen based on the desire to move the implant interface away from the bone in a vertical direction. Since the implants were to be placed in completely regenerated bone, a tissue-level prosthetic connection was used to protect the marginal bone levels over the long term. There is ample evidence supporting the long-term stability of this type of implants (Jung and coworkers 2013; Buser and coworkers 2012). The follow-up situation showed stable clinical and radiographic results two and ten years after delivery, with esthetically pleasing crowns.

Prosthetic rehabilitation. All-ceramic crowns on implants have yielded high survival rates comparable to those of metal-ceramic reconstructions (Raigrodski and coworkers 2012; Sailer and coworkers 2015), and they commonly achieve high levels of esthetic patient satisfaction (Buchi and coworkers 2014; Thoma and coworkers 2016). The two implants in this case were restored with all-ceramic individual crowns on In-Ceram abutments and with a feldspathic ceramic veneer, a technique that has also provided high long-term survival rates (Fenner and coworkers 2016). The patient was very satisfied with the esthetic result of the implant crowns, which have not presented any complications in more than ten years.

6.7 Early Implant Placement, Contour Augmentation, and Autologous Connective-Tissue Graft Using a Tunneling Technique to Replace an Upper Incisor with Generalized Gingival Recession

E. Lorenzana, J. Gillespie

Variations in soft-tissue volume, evidenced either by an overabundance (Evian and coworkers 1993; Levine and McGuire1997; Dolt and Robbins 1997) or by a deficiency of soft or hard tissue can complicate implant-supported rehabilitations in the esthetic zone (Lorenzana 2008; Lorenzana and coworkers 2009). The present case illustrates the replacement of a failing upper left lateral incisor complicated by generalized severe gingival recession in the esthetic zone.

Presenting complaint

A healthy 66-year-old woman was referred for a consultation to evaluate the replacement of tooth 22 with an implant-supported restoration. The patient reported a history of previous endodontic treatment on tooth 22 and multiple class V composite restorations provided to address gingival recessions throughout the anterior sextant. The tooth had recently fractured and was deemed non-restorable by her restorative dentist (Dr. Jason Gillespie), who had temporarily bonded tooth 22 to the

adjacent teeth to immobilize the fractured segment. The patient was subsequently referred for evaluation for an implant-supported restoration at site 22 and treatment of multiple gingival recessions on the maxillary and mandibular anterior teeth. A review of her anamnesis yielded a history of breast cancer and controlled hypertension, with no known drug allergies.

The patient presented with excellent oral hygiene (full-mouth plaque score under 10%), and the full-mouth probing chart did not reveal any pockets deeper than 4 mm.

Analysis of her smile revealed a medium, symmetrical smile line, with only the interdental papillae visible at full smile. In addition, mild crowding was evident, with tooth 21 slightly overlapping tooth 11. The patient expressed no interest in orthodontic therapy. Tooth 22 was discolored and slightly displaced following its fracture (Fig 1).

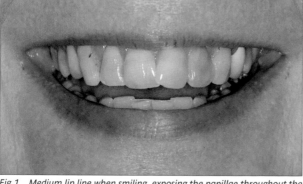

Fig 1   Medium lip line when smiling, exposing the papillae throughout the anterior sextant. Upper lip obscuring the gingival margins of the central incisors.

The anterior retracted view revealed a thin gingival phenotype with triangular-shaped teeth and elongated papillae (Fig 2). Discoloration of tooth 22 was evident, together with a thin band of attached gingiva bordering the multiple gingival recessions affecting teeth 13 to 23. Teeth 13, 22, and 23 had class V bonded composite restorations, where the recessions measured from 3 to 5 mm across the maxillary and mandibular sextants.

A focused view of tooth 22 more clearly illustrated the lack of soft tissue on the buccal aspect and the continued retraction of the gingival margin past the margin of the class V restoration (Fig 3). Such an observation indicates ongoing recession. In an intact dentition, this situation should be treated by augmenting the gingival volume and addressing the factors contributing to the progression of the recession, including occlusal trauma, destructive hygiene habits, or inadequate restorative interventions.

The initial periapical radiograph of tooth 22 revealed a silver-point endodontic restoration within a long root and a clearly visible fracture line. In addition, the root of tooth 22 was not centered within the proposed implant site, being instead close to tooth 12. Finally, a distal curve at the apical end of the root was visible, indicating a potentially complicated extraction (Fig 4).

The patient was referred for a preoperative cone-beam computed tomography (CBCT) that demonstrated an adequate base of bone apical and palatal to the root apex to allow engagement of the native alveolar bone by the implant following the extraction of the tooth (Fig 5). However, the buccal bone plate was not visible until approximately midway down the root, corroborating the advanced gingival recession observed clinically. Finally, the CBCT indicated possible internal root resorption of tooth 22.

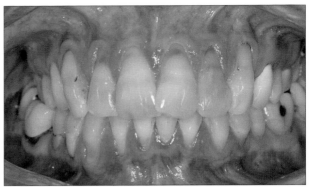

Fig 2   Retracted view. Thin gingival phenotype with generalized maxillary and mandibular gingival recessions.

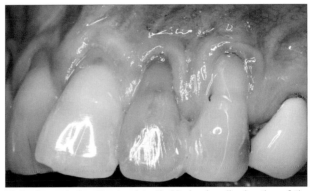

Fig 3   Focused view. Fractured tooth 22 showing discoloration of the tooth, 4.5 mm of recession and a class V composite restoration.

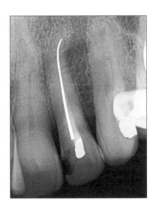

Fig 4   Periapical radiograph. Fracture extent and previous endodontic treatment with a silver-point filling and apical root curvature.

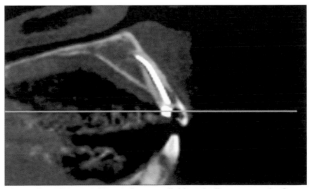

Fig 5   CBCT image. Adequate bone available apically to secure the fixture but with 50% buccal bone loss.

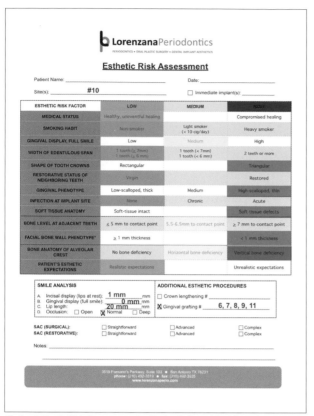

Fig 6 Esthetic Risk Assessment, Smile Analysis and SAC form in use at the author's private practice.

A complete risk assessment was performed using a customized Esthetic Risk Assessment form. This form incorporates the recently updated Esthetic Risk Assessment table (Martin and coworkers 2017) as well as a brief smile analysis, the expected additional esthetic procedures that could impact the implant position or the overall esthetic outcome, and, finally, assignment of the appropriate SAC level (Fig 6). Upon completion, this form was shared with the patient and the restorative team.

Multiple elevated risk factors were identified, including triangular-shaped teeth, a thin phenotype, soft-tissue defects, a facial bone wall phenotype of less than 1 mm thickness, and a vertical bone deficiency along the buccal aspect due to the gingival recession. A medium lip line and expected horizontal extraction defect contributed to the medium risk factors. Gingival grafting of teeth 13, 12, 11, 21, and 23 was expected. Finally, the patient was assigned complex surgical and advanced restorative SAC classifications.

Fig 7 illustrates the desired treatment outcome by outlining the ideal gingival margin positions of teeth 13 to 23. By establishing the goal of a more ideal, coronally positioned augmented gingival margin, the desired three-dimensional implant position 3 to 3.5 mm apical to the desired new gingival margin can then be determined.

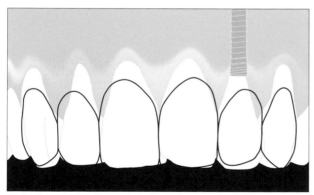

Fig 7 Crown dimension outlines. Desired outcome following treatment. Implant shoulder was positioned 3 to 3.5 mm apical to the desired gingival margin.

Treatment options

Several treatment options were considered to create the desired result, including:

1. Extraction of tooth 22 with ridge preservation site 22, plus simultaneous autologous connective-tissue grafting of adjacent sites 13 – 23
2. Extraction of tooth 22 with collagen plug placement, healing for six to eight weeks, followed by early (Type 2) implant placement, GBR and autologous or allogeneic connective-tissue grafting of the adjacent sites 13 – 23
3. Orthodontic extrusion of tooth 22, followed by immediate implant placement, GBR and autologous or allogeneic connective-tissue grafting
4. Extraction of tooth 22 with ridge preservation, simultaneous autologous connective-tissue grafting of the adjacent dentition 13 – 23, and fabrication of a fixed partial denture or Maryland bridge

While all four options are reasonable, Option 3 could be immediately discarded, since the patient had stated at the initial visit that orthodontic treatment was not an option for her. Of the remaining possibilities, Option 2 was chosen because it could be completed within a shorter time frame.

Tooth 22 was removed using minimally traumatic techniques to preserve the soft tissue and surrounding alveolar bone (Fig 8). Briefly, a powered periotome (Powertome 100S, Westport Medical), was utilized to separate the tooth from the alveolus, then the tooth was delivered with traditional forceps. Following atraumatic extraction of the tooth, a collagen plug was placed within the socket and secured with a 5-0 chromic gut suture (Ethicon, Somerville, NJ, USA). No incisions and no tissue trauma or displacement were present following extraction. The root was sectioned from tooth 22 and the crown was bonded to the adjacent teeth as a provisional restoration during the healing phase.

Six weeks after the extraction, the soft tissues at site 22 were completely healed and healthy, with most of the previously observed recession defect resolved. The patient was at this point deemed ready to proceed with implant placement, GBR, and soft-tissue augmentation (Fig 9).

The bonded provisional restoration was removed to expose site 22 prior to surgery (Fig 10). The tissues were confirmed to be healthy, with a significant gain in volume that would allow for primary closure after the surgical procedure.

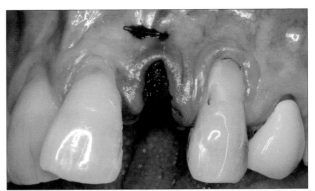

Fig 8 Tooth 22 removed with collagen plug in place.

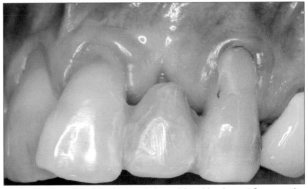

Fig 9 Healing of site 22 with bonded provisional in place at four months.

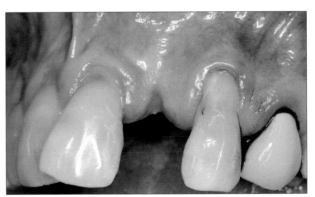

Fig 10 Site 22 prior to surgery. Complete epithelialization of site 22 at four months, ready for implant placement and GBR.

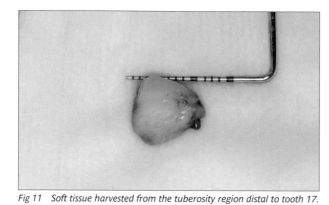

Fig 11   Soft tissue harvested from the tuberosity region distal to tooth 17.

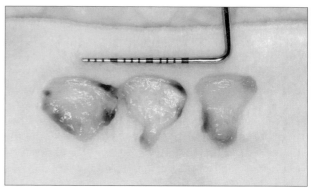

Fig 12   Tuberosity graft sectioned into three 1- to 1.5-mm sections.

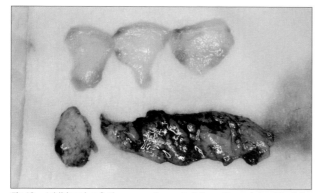

Fig 13   Additional soft tissue was harvested from the palate. All of the harvested soft tissue is shown.

Figures 11 and 12 show the tissue harvested from the tuberosity distal to tooth 27 followed by careful sectioning of the tissue to create ideal tissue-graft thickness of 1 to 1.5 mm.

Additional tissue was obtained from the left palatal vault through a single-incision technique (Lorenzana and Allen 2000). The total tissue harvested is shown in Fig 13.

Following reflection of a full-thickness flap, an implant (Bone Level Narrow CrossFit, diameter 3.3 mm, length 14 mm; Institut Straumann AG, Basel, Switzerland) was placed in the correct three-dimensional position as planned, with the implant shoulder positioned 3 mm away from the gingival margin (Figs 14 and 15).

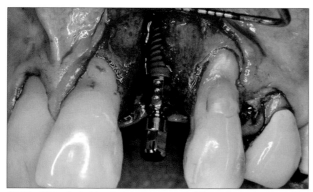

Fig 14   The selected implant in the corrected three-dimensional position before GBR and soft-tissue grafting.

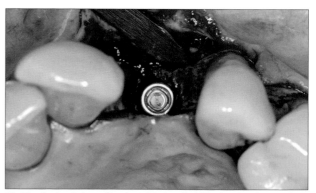

Fig 15   Occlusal view of implant 22 placed within the alveolar envelope, on the palatal aspect of the alveolar socket.

Specialized tunneling instruments were employed to elevate the tissue (Allen End-Cutting Intrasulcular Knife, Allen Periosteal Elevator Anterior, and Allen Arrowhead Knife; Hu-Friedy, Chicago, IL, USA), creating a tunnel-bed preparation from tooth 13 to 21 (Fig 16). A periodontal probe was used to verify the continuity of the tunnel preparation.

The larger connective-tissue graft was carefully guided into the tunnel and secured with circumferential 5-0 chromic gut sutures over teeth 13 to 21 (Fig 17). Additional soft tissue was secured over tooth 23 in a similar manner. GBR was then performed over implant 22 in the manner reported by Buser and coworkers (2008), with autologous bone chips placed over the implant followed by xenograft derived from deproteinized bovine bone mineral (Bio-Oss; Geistlich, Wolhusen, Switzerland). Finally, a dual layer of non-crosslinked collagen membrane (Bio-Gide; Geistlich) was applied over the bone grafts.

Flap closure was accomplished with 6-0 monofilament nylon suture (Ethilon; Ethicon) applied as sling sutures over the soft-tissue grafting sites, and horizontal mattress and interrupted sutures over the GBR site (Fig 18). With the extra soft tissue created following removal of tooth 22 during the early healing phase, tension-free primary closure was more easily achieved.

The postoperative radiograph confirmed the ideal position of the dental implant, away from the adjacent roots and any vital structures (Fig 19).

The two-week follow-up photograph illustrates uneventful healing, with complete root coverage already evident at the soft-tissue grafting sites (Fig 20). A bonded provisional restoration was once more employed during the healing phase.

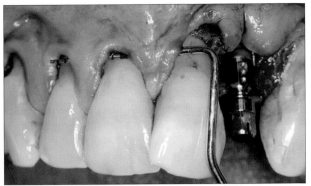

Fig 16 *Completed tunnel preparation. Continuity verified with a periodontal probe within the tunnel.*

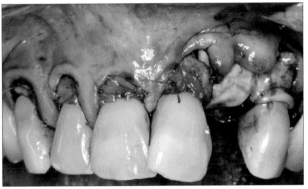

Fig 17 *Completed GBR procedures. Soft-tissue grafts in place.*

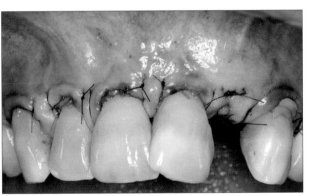

Fig 18 *Completed closure of the surgical site.*

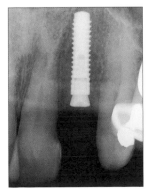

Fig 19 *Radiograph taken immediately at the end of the procedure, confirming the implant position.*

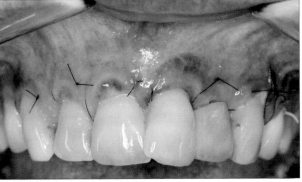

Fig 20 *Two-week postoperative situation. Excellent healing and adaptation of the soft tissues.*

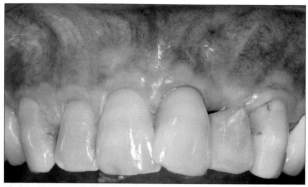

Fig 21   Four-month situation. Tissue maturation prior to uncovering.

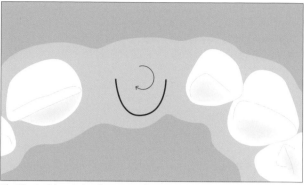

Fig 22   Incision design for uncovering.

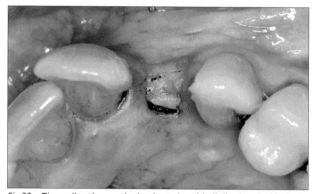

Fig 23   Tissue directly over the implant, de-epithelialized and with the incision completed.

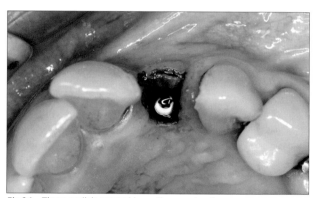

Fig 24   Tissue pedicle rotated buccally, exposing the cover screw.

At four months, the soft tissues had matured and the implant was ready for uncovering (Fig 21). Although an adequate band of keratinized mucosa was already present, uncovering of the implant provides an additional opportunity to create additional soft-tissue volume on the buccal aspect of the implant in preparation for provisionalization and tissue shaping.

A U-shaped incision design was used over the implant to create a pedicle of soft tissue that can be displaced facially (Barone and coworkers 1999; Mühlemann and coworkers 2012). This pedicle graft was then displaced facially into a shallow pouch that was then secured with a healing cap and sutures (Fig 22).

The occlusal view of the implant site illustrates the need for additional buccal soft-tissue volume (Fig 23). First, the U-shaped incision was made and the overlying tissue de-epithelialized using a fine No. 8 diamond round bur (Brasseler, Savannah, GA, USA).

The tissue was elevated with an Orban knife, exposing the healing abutment (diameter 3.6 mm, height 2 mm) (Fig 24). The tissue was carefully tucked into the buccal aspect with a tunneling instrument (Allen Periosteal Elevator Anterior; Hu-Friedy).

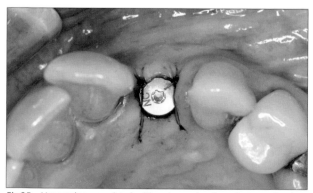

Fig 25   Uncovering completed with a larger healing abutment in place and sutures to secure the flap.

The original healing cap was replaced with another healing abutment (diameter 4.8 mm, height 5 mm) to help position the rotated pedicle flap (Fig 25). Additional 5-0 chromic gut sutures were applied to further secure the area.

A provisional restoration was fabricated and delivered to initiate shaping of the peri-implant tissues (Fig 26). A follow-up radiograph was also taken at this time to verify stable bone levels around the implant (Fig 27).

A digital impression was taken. A customized zirconia abutment was designed and fabricated using CARES (Straumann). The abutment was torqued to 35 Ncm (Fig 28).

A custom stained and glazed lithium disilicate crown was fabricated and cemented using a radiopaque luting agent (IPS e.max; Ivoclar Vivadent, Schaan, Liechtenstein; and MaxCem; Kerr Dental, Orange, USA). Figure 29 shows the final restoration on the day of delivery.

The photograph taken at the three-year follow-up demonstrated stable, symmetric tissue contours, with gingival margins free of inflammation or other complications (Fig 30).

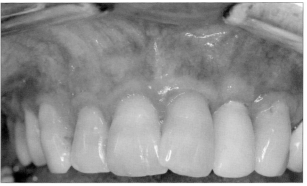

Fig 26   Provisional restoration in place.

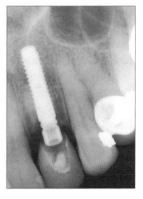

Fig 27   Follow-up radiograph with provisional in place documenting healing of the fixture.

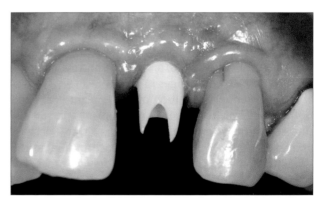

Fig 28   The customized CARES abutment in situ.

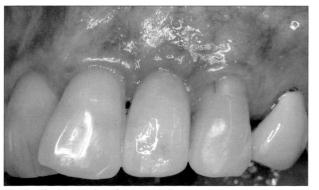

Fig 29   Final restoration after cementation.

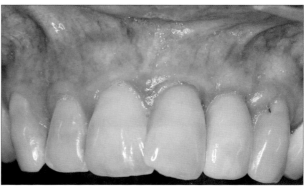

Fig 30   Retracted anterior view at three years. Well-maintained soft-tissue profile.

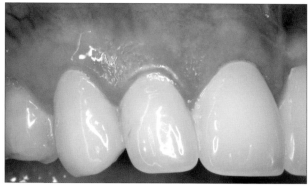

Fig 3   Contour of the restored natural tooth.

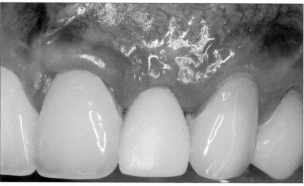

Fig 4   Contour of implant 22 provisional crown. Side-by-side comparison highlighting the lack of symmetry in the emergence profile.

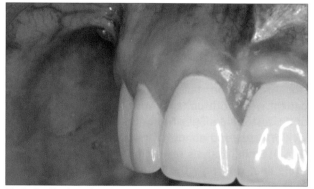

Fig 5   Profile view of tooth 12.

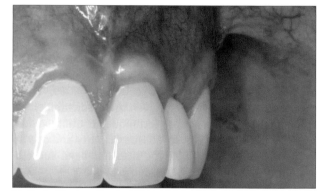

Fig 6   Profile view of implant 22 highlighting the lack of soft-tissue volume.

Although the implant appeared to be in the ideal three-dimensional position, the lack of symmetry between tooth 12 and 22 was evident, with a deficient apical third of the restoration at the gingival margin.

Side-by-side comparison of 12 and 22 more clearly illustrated the lack of symmetry in crown form and contour caused by the lack of buccal tissue volume (Figs 3 and 4). Furthermore, the crown margin at 21 and 23 was exposed and visible (Fig 4).

A look at the long axes of tooth 12 and implant 22 further underscored the atypical emergence profile of implant 22 due to the lack of soft-tissue volume (Figs 5 and 6).

Fig 7 illustrates how the lack of tissue support resulted in an inadequate cervical contour of the restoration. It was recommended to add connective tissue to the buccal aspect of site 22 and to recontour the provisional to the desired shape and emergence profile (Fig 7).

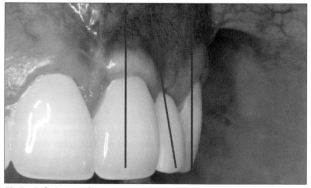

Fig 7   Soft-tissue deficiency on the buccal aspect of implant 22 impacting the angle of emergence of the restoration.

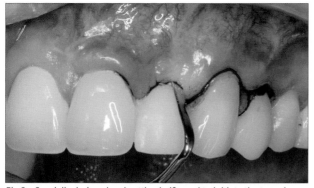

Fig 8   Specially designed end-cutting knife used to initiate the tunnel preparation.

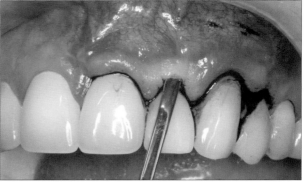

Fig 9   Tissue carefully elevated with a specially designed tunneling elevator.

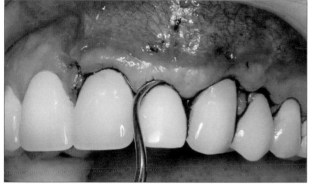

Fig 10   Elevation of the papillae and release of remaining tissue tags with a curved periodontal universal curette.

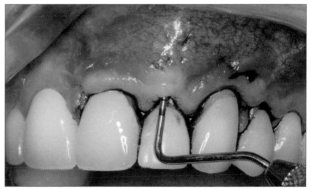

Fig 11   Periodontal probe demonstrating the depth of the pouch preparation.

The initial incision was made using a specially designed end-cutting knife (Allen End-Cutting Intrasulcular Knife; Hu-Friedy, Chicago, IL, USA) along the buccal and distobuccal aspect of tooth 21, the buccal and mesiobuccal aspect of tooth 23, and circumferentially around implant 22. The incision was further extended across the papilla distal to tooth 23. This incision design would allow for maximum elevation and release of the tissue coronally (Fig 8).

The tissue was elevated with a specially designed tunneling elevator that allows for blunt dissection of the tissue

pouch, minimizing perforations or tears (Allen Periosteal Elevator Anterior; Hu-Friedy) (Fig 9).

A universal periodontal scaler with a rounded blade edge (Younger-Good 7/8; Hu-Friedy) was used to elevate the interdental papillae and finish releasing tissue tags within the tunnel preparation (Fig 10).

Finally, a periodontal probe was used to verify the continuity of the tunnel preparation and that the pouch was ready to accommodate the connective-tissue graft (Figs 11 and 12).

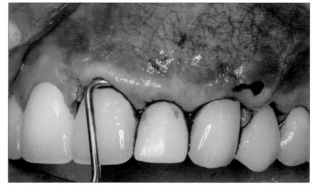

Fig 12   Continuity of the tunnel preparation verified with the periodontal probe.

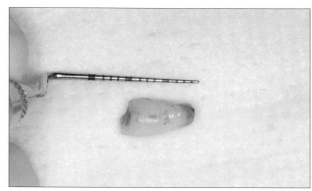

Fig 13   Graft as initially harvested from the tuberosity.

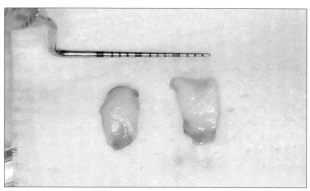

Fig 14   Final grafts shaped prior to delivery.

The traditional donor site for connective tissue tends to be the palatal vault (Langer and Langer 1985; Lorenzana and Allen 2000). However, alternative donor sites exist, with the most common secondary donor site being the tuberosity region distal to the maxillary second molars (Studer and coworkers 1997). Advantages of this donor site include the remote location away from the tongue, the increased density of the tissue, and the reported lower morbidity and pain (Rojo and coworkers 2018; Amin and coworkers 2018; Godat and coworkers 2018). A recent histological study found increased lamina propia vs. submucosa in tuberosity grafts compared to palatal grafts, which the authors concluded could prove beneficial when performing volume augmentation (Sanz-Martín and coworkers 2018).

The patient presented with adequate donor tissue in the tuberosity region distal to tooth 27. Figures 13 and 14 show the tissue harvested from the area, followed by the careful sectioning of the tissue to obtain the desired graft thickness of approximately 2 mm for site 22. The additional soft tissue was to be placed at tooth 23.

With a periodontal probe acting as a retractor, a 5-0 chromic gut suture (Ethicon; Somerville, NJ, USA) was introduced into the apical aspect of the pouch and exited through the coronal aspect of the tunnel preparation (Fig 15).

Next, the intended apical aspect of the connective-tissue graft was made to engage with the suture and the needle reinserted into the pouch and out of the apical aspect of the tunnel. This allowed the suture to guide the graft into the pouch and secure it apically (Fig 16).

Figure 17 demonstrates the graft being guided into the pouch through the sulcus.

Finally, the tissue graft was secured coronally with a circumferential 5-0 chromic gut suture. The extra soft tissue was placed at tooth 23 (Fig 18).

Circumferential 6-0 nylon sutures (Ethicon) were used to coronally advance and secure the tissue flap (Fig 19).

The view along the axis of implant 22 illustrates the amount of volume augmentation achieved (Fig 20).

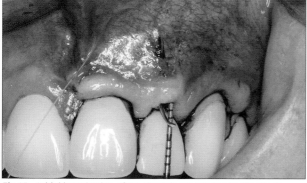

Fig 15   Initial introduction of the chromic gut suture into the pouch.

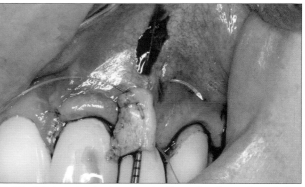

Fig 16   5-0 chromic gut suture engaging the graft and emerging apically.

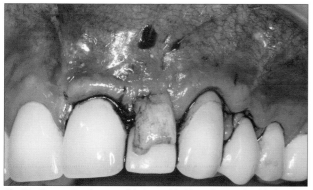

Fig 17   Connective-tissue graft being guided into the pouch with the chromic gut suture.

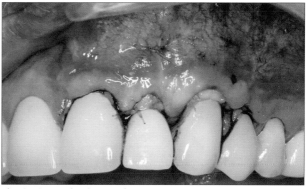

Fig 18   Connective-tissue grafts secured within the tunnel preparation.

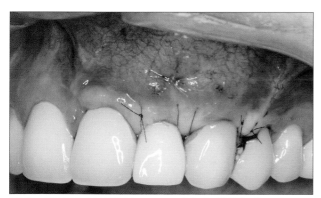

Fig 19   Final suturing of the area accomplished with 6-0 nylon sutures.

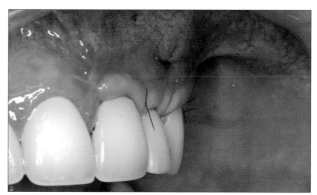

Fig 20   View along the axis of implant 22 demonstrating the amount of volume augmentation achieved.

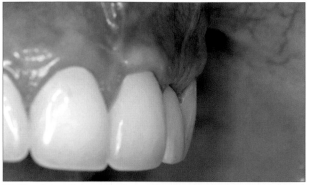

Fig 21   Five-week postoperative profile view of implant 22 showing excellent healing and volume gain.

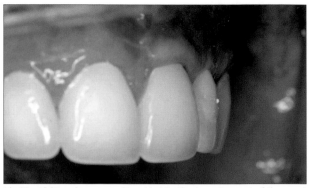

Fig 22   Light-curing composite added to the buccal aspect of the provisional crown to define the desired emergence profile.

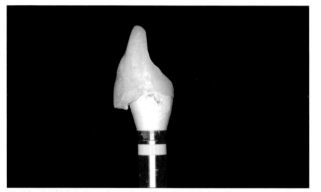

Fig 23   Provisional on the NC analog showing the discrepancy between the crown contour and the provisional abutment margin.

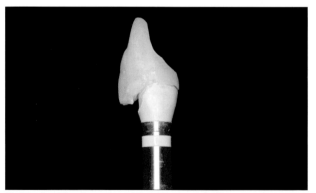

Fig 24   Provisional margin positioned further apically.

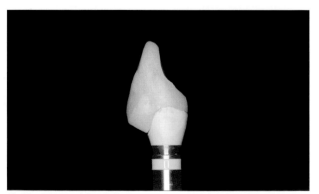

Fig 25   New provisional abutment and complete crown contours.

Five weeks after the augmentation, the volume attained was evident (Fig 21), so that provisional reshaping could be initiated.

The first step in this process was to create the desired final crown contour with composite resin prior to removing the provisional (Fig 22).

Upon removal of the provisional crown and abutment, the discrepancy between the desired emergence profile and the provisional abutment margin was evident (Narrow CrossFit PEEK; Institut Straumann AG, Basel, Switzerland) (Fig 23).

Next, the abutment was re-prepared to create a more apical finish line (Fig 24). This allowed for a smoother transition from the abutment to the height of contour at the gingival zenith. In this case, a modifiable PEEK plastic provisional abutment was utilized. Another option would have been to use a one-piece screw-retained provisional crown for tissue shaping. This would have eliminated any cement finish line that may cause irritation to the tissues.

The completed provisional abutment and crown were now ready for delivery (Fig 25).

Figure 26 shows the provisional in place following soft-tissue augmentation and recontouring of the provisional abutment and crown.

Viewing the provisional restoration along the long axis of the tooth revealed significant improvement in soft-tissue volume and the improved emergence profile (Fig 27).

The patient was delighted by the improvement in her smile and agreed to now proceed to the final restoration (Fig 28).

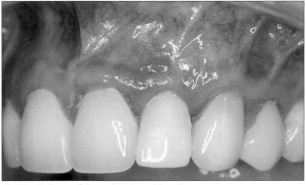

Fig 26   Delivery of the updated provisional.

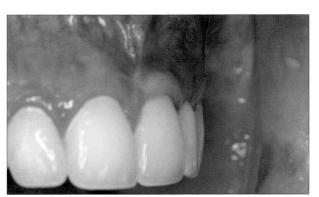

Fig 27   Profile view showing the desired emergence profile and tissue support.

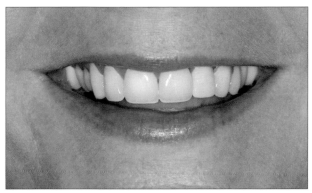

Fig 28   The patient was now pleased with her smile.

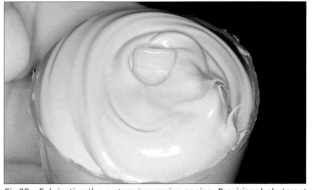

Fig 29   Fabricating the custom impression coping. Provisional abutment and crown on an NC analog, immersed in bite-registration material.

To accurately transfer the emergence profile to the master cast for the fabrication of the final restoration, a custom impression coping was made (Figs 29 to 31). First, the provisional abutment and crown were removed and seated on a Narrow CrossFit analog. After applying petroleum jelly to the abutment and crown, bite registration material (Blu-Mousse; Parkell, Edgewood, NY, USA) was applied around the provisional and allowed to set (Fig 29). The buccal aspect was marked with a red permanent marker for reference. The provisional crown and abutment were removed, leaving an outline of the emergence profile (Fig 30). A Bone Level NC impression post was placed into the mold, then composite material was slowly added to fill the voids around the impression post and light-cured until set (Fig 31).

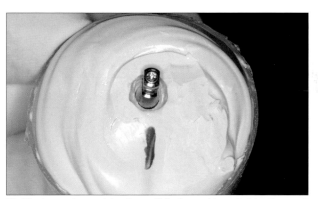

Fig 30   Impression post in place within the mold created by the provisional.

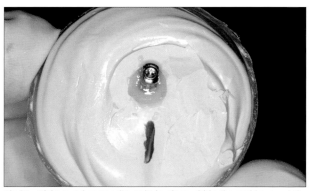

Fig 31   Light-cured composite resin in place within the mold around the impression post.

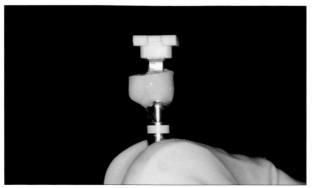

Fig 32   Final custom impression post.

The final custom impression post was now ready for impression-taking (Fig 32).

The custom impression post was marked on the buccal aspect to ensure proper orientation before being seated in the mouth (Figs 33 and 34). Because the shape of the coping was identical to the provisional, it preserved support for the tissues during the impression procedures, thus transferring to the laboratory the desired shape for the final restoration.

Figures 35 and 36 show the final one-piece screw-retained metal-ceramic restoration three years after delivery. The tissues were stable and free of inflammation and complications.

The three-year photograph of the final restoration in profile demonstrate the maintenance of the soft-tissue volume obtained thanks to the connective-tissue graft (Fig 37).

The three-year photograph of the patient's smile clearly illustrated her satisfaction with the esthetic result (Fig 38).

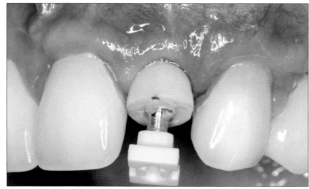

Fig 33   Custom impression post in place, buccal view.

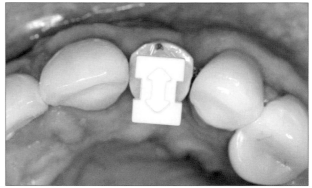

Fig 34   Occlusal view. Custom impression post in place.

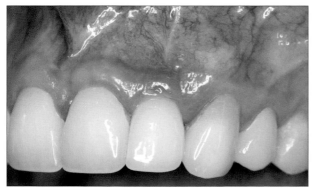

Fig 35   Final restoration at three years.

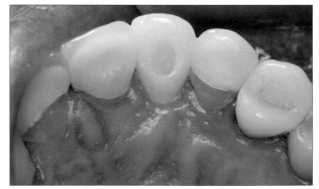

Fig 36   Occlusal view. Final screw-retained restoration.

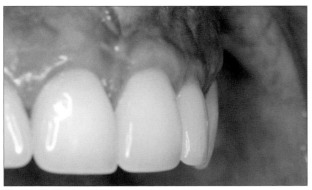

Fig 37 Profile view at three years.

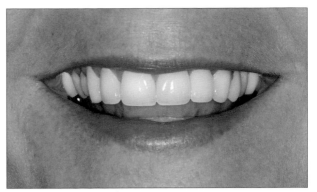

Fig 38 Patient's smile at three years.

Stable bone levels were evident around the implant in the four-year radiograph; the emergence profile of the final restoration was in harmony with the bone profile at the implant site (Fig 39).

Discussion

Biological, technical, or esthetic complications can occur during any stage of the implant-based reconstructive process. In the case presented here, it was fortuitous that the issue was identified prior to delivery of the final prosthesis, because modifications to the restoration and additional surgical reconstructive procedures are simpler to accomplish during the provisional phase than with a final prosthesis in place. Furthermore, there was no recession of the marginal tissue around the implant to complicate the situation.

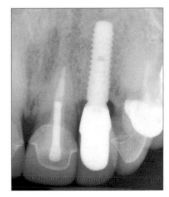

Fig 39 Periapical radiograph at four years.

With the implant in an ideal three-dimensional position, the chief complaint from the patient and referring dentist was the lack of tissue volume on the buccal aspect of the implant, resulting in an inadequate emergence profile of the provisional restoration. There are many case reports in the literature describing connective-tissue grafts to augment the soft-tissue volume around implants (Silverstein and Lefkove 1994; Akcalı and coworkers 2015). Connective-tissue grafting techniques continue to be the preferred method of augmenting the soft-tissue volume around teeth and implants (Thoma and coworkers 2009, 2014; Levine and coworkers 2014).

From a practical standpoint, reducing invasiveness and morbidity during these procedures is important to the patient and clinician. Tunneling and alternative harvesting techniques have been developed to aid in achieving this goal (Allen 1994; Lorenzana and Allen 2000; Godat and coworkers 2018). In this case, a tunneling approach to site preparation was employed together with soft tissue harvested from the tuberosity region of the maxilla.

As mentioned previously, the location of the donor site away from the tongue, the increased density of the tissue, and reported lower morbidity and pain are all advantages of tuberosity donor sites. This yielded the required volume augmentation resulting in the desired esthetic and functional result.

Although recent literature reviews have documented a lack of controlled clinical trials for these types of situations, numerous case series and case reports such as the one presented here cast a positive light on the application of these techniques. Further study with long-term controlled clinical trials is recommended.

Acknowledgments

Restorative procedures
Kurt Riewe, DDS – San Antonio, TX, USA

Laboratory procedures
3D Ceramics – San Antonio, TX, USA

6.9 Treatment of Soft-Tissue Fenestration in the Esthetic Zone

N. MacBeth, N. Donos

Presenting complaint

A 42-year-old man presented with a swelling adjacent to an implant crown at site 21. The swelling had been present for approximately three weeks and was constrained to the buccal and palatal gingival aspects of the implant. A discharge was noted on finger pressure, with localized gingival recession present on the mid- and distolabial aspects of the crown.

The patient had experienced one episode of swelling approximately four months previously, with localized exudate noted from the buccal and palatal aspects of the implant crown on this occasion. The inflammation had partially resolved following subgingival debridement of the area, but progressive gingival recession had been noted over a successive six-month period, with a draining sinus now present 3 mm below the gingival margin (Figs 1a-c).

The patient had not experienced any pain or discomfort from the area but was worried that the presence of infection at the implant site would result in bone loss around the implant fixture, jeopardizing the long-term survival of the implant. He was also concerned about the degree of recession present at sites 21 and 22, as the tissue loss was visible, affecting his confidence when smiling.

The implant had been placed in 2004, following the loss of the tooth due to endodontic complications. A replacement implant-supported crown had been provided in 2011, following localized trauma to the area. Gingival recession around the implant crown had been first charted in 2013, with no record of progressive attachment loss or additional gingival recession around teeth 21 to 24 over the next five years.

The patient present with no relevant medical history, no current medication, and no known allergies. He was a non-smoker and had an occasional nocturnal parafunctional grinding habit. He reported a pen-chewing habit on the anterior dentition when at work.

He was a regular dental attender who underwent yearly periodontal maintenance following a diagnosis of localized periodontitis (stage II/grade A) in the molar areas and peri-implant mucositis around the implant-supported crown 21.

His current oral-hygiene regime included the use of an electric toothbrush twice daily, with occasional use of interproximal TePe brushes (TePe Munhygienprodukter, Malmö, Sweden). He had been advised to use an electric toothbrush to reduce the risks of trauma from abrasion by a manual toothbrush.

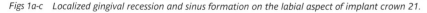

Figs 1a-c   Localized gingival recession and sinus formation on the labial aspect of implant crown 21.

N. MacBeth, N. Donos

Preoperative examination and diagnosis

At the clinical examination, the patient presented with a class 1 skeletal base, no lymphadenopathy, TMJ abnormality, crepitus, or limitation in his range of jaw movement.

The intraoral examination revealed the presence of a prominent linea alba on the left buccal mucosa, with the tongue and oral tissues pink and healthy.

Gingival inflammation was noted around implant crown 21, presenting as a red and edematous peri-implant gingival collar, with discharge from the buccal and palatal margins on digital pressure and a localized draining sinus, 3 mm below the mid-gingival margin of crown 21.

A full-mouth pocket chart recorded probing pocket depths of 3 mm on the mesio-, mid- and distolabial surfaces of the implant crown and of 5 mm on the corresponding palatal surfaces (Fig 2). No plaque or calculus deposits were detected at the crown/abutment interface, but bleeding on probing was elicited from the buccal and palatal gingival margins. The full-mouth plaque score (FMPS) was 3% and the full-mouth bleeding score (FMBS) was 4%. Pockets of more than 3 mm were detected at sites 21, 27, 28, 37, and 38. Generalized recession was present throughout the mouth, with a review of the clinical records first indicating localized gingival recession around implant crown 21 in 2013. The gingival tissue level had then stabilized over the subsequent six months, with no further attachment loss recorded over the next five years (Fig 3).

Examination of the dentition revealed the presence of a cemented Nobel Procera crown 21 with a custom zirconia abutment. A small marginal gap was present between the crown and the abutment, in the palatal area. Indirect cast-gold restorations were present on teeth 36 and 46, with evidence of tooth surface loss seen on teeth 16–11, 22–26, 32–35, and 41–45. The surface loss was principally confined to the incisal aspects of the anterior dentition and the buccal aspects of the premolar and molar teeth (Fig 4).

Occlusal examination revealed a class 1 occlusal scheme, with normal overjet and overbite. Canine guidance was present in right and left lateral excursions, with even contact present between the maxillary and mandibular incisors on protrusive movements. No evidence of loosening was recorded for crown 21.

REC (B)		132	101	222	122	221	121	000		133	343	133	222	222	233	100	000
PPD (P)		333	332	223	222	222	222	222		555	222	222	322	222	333	534	434
PPD (B)		333	223	222	222	322	223	322		333	222	222	322	223	333	435	534
Tooth position		17	16	15	14	13	12	11		21	22	23	24	25	26	27	28
Tooth position		47	46	45	44	43	42	41		31	32	33	34	35	36	37	38
PPD (B)		333	322	222	222	322	222	222		222	222	222	222	323	233	433	333
PPD (L)		333	323	222	222	222	222	222		222	222	222	223	322	333	434	433
REC (B)		001	000	121	122	221	000	021		000	021	232	232	222	110	000	000

Fig 2   Full-mouth pocket chart recorded at emergency appointment.

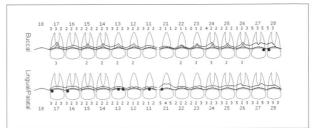

Fig 3   Maxillary pocket chart taken six months prior to presentation.

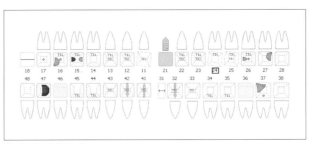

Fig 4   Dental chart.

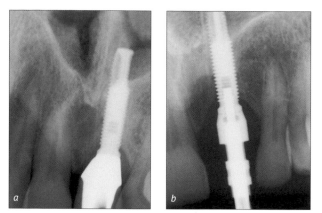

Figs 5a-b   Radiograph of the implant fixture at the time of crown replacement and at the consultation appointment.

An intraoral radiograph of site 21 indicated the presence of an implant (Brånemark MK-III TiUnite, diameter 3.75 mm, length 18 mm; Nobel Biocare, Kloten, Switzerland), with the implant fixture extending through the nasal floor. Coronally, the alveolar bone level was based at the second thread of the implant on the mesial aspect and the first thread on the distal aspect. Comparison with previous radiographs indicated no progressive bone loss after the crown had been replaced 5 years previously (Figs 5a-b). Bitewing radiographs indicated horizontal bone loss of 1 to 2 mm in the molar areas.

Diagnosis

The following diagnoses were made:

- Peri-implant mucositis, implant 21
- Localized periodontitis, stage II, grade A, currently stable

- Abutment-level abscess with draining sinus, associated with the presence of a marginal discrepancy at the crown 21/abutment interface
- Tooth surface loss attributed to parafunctional attrition (mild)

Treatment plan

Stabilization phase:

- Oral-hygiene reinforcement, with emphasis on interdental and marginal cleaning of implant site 21 and the molar areas
- Debridement of the maxillary right posterior region
- Local debridement of the coronal collar of the implant and irrigation of the site according to Cumulative Interceptive Supportive Therapy (CIST) protocol (Lang and coworkers 2004)
- Recording of FMPS and FMBS at each visit to review the patient's motivation and oral hygiene
- Repeated pocket and recession charts at six months
- Removal of implant-supported crown and abutment and placement of a cover screw on implant 21 to promote healing of the gingival tissue and closure over cover screw 21

Regenerative phase:

- Placement of a subepithelial connective-tissue graft at site 21/22 in conjunction with a coronally advanced flap to augment the gingival tissue around implant 21 and tooth 22 (Bassetti and coworkers 2017)
- Exposure of the implant following three months of healing
- Correction of the emergence profile of the implant crown to reduce the loss of interproximal papillary tissue
- Review to determine the need for additional periodontal grafting to cover the recession defect

Long-term maintenance:

- Periodontal review at six and twelve months to monitor the peri-implant gingival status and tooth attachment levels
- Radiographic review of site 21 and the maxillary left quadrant at twelve months
- Reinforcement of oral hygiene, including interdental cleaning, with additional periodontal cause-related therapy if required

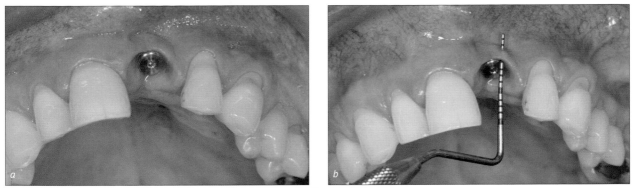

Figs 6a-b   Gingival healing at two weeks, following removal of the prosthetic superstructure.

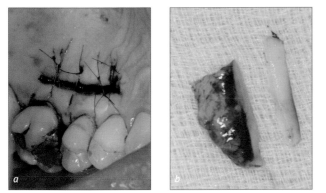

Figs 7a-b   Connective tissue harvested from the palatal region.

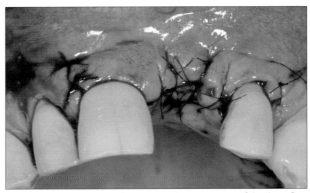

Fig 8   Connective-tissue graft and coronal advancement of the tissue flap.

Treatment procedures

The initial treatment consisted of localized subgingival debridement in the maxillary right posterior region and reinforcement of the patient's oral hygiene. The interdental cleaning regime was emphasized, using Oral-B Superfloss (Procter & Gamble, Weybridge, UK) and TePe brushes (TePe Munhygienprodukter) in the molar areas.

As the marginal defect was present at the crown-abutment junction, it was felt that removal of the implant crown and prosthetic abutment would eliminate the bacterial contamination, allowing resolution of the chronic infection at this site. The prosthetic crown was therefore sectioned to allow access to the retaining screw; after removal, a cover screw was placed to encourage tissue growth over the implant fixture (Figs 6a-b). Non-surgical debridement of the coronal neck of the implant surface was undertaken under local anesthesia using titanium implant scalers (Hu-Friedy, Chicago, IL, USA) and rubber polishing cups. The crown was replaced with a provisional maxillary partial acrylic denture (Every design), with the pontic shaped to preserve the interproximal papillary structure.

A 18 × 10 mm connective-tissue graft was harvested from the palatal aspect of site 14 – 16 according to the technique described by Bruno (1994) (Figs 7a-b). The epithelial layer was then removed from the donor tissue prior to preparation of the recipient site.

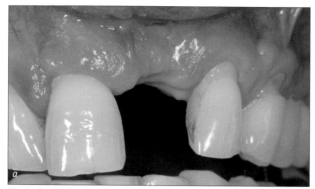

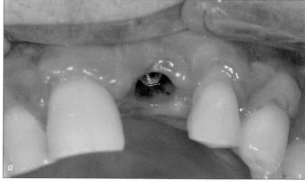

Figs 9a-b   Grafted implant site at twelve weeks.

Figs 10a-b   Increase in gingival peri-implant collar thickness at the fixture-level impression appointment.

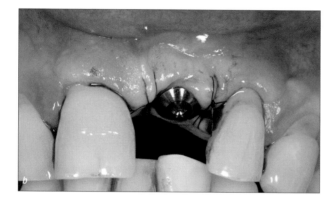

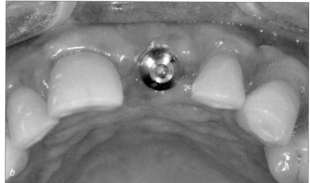

A full-thickness trapezoidal flap was raised to the level of the mucogingival junction. A partial-thickness flap was dissected beyond the mucogingival junction, leaving the underlying alveolar bone covered with periosteum and connective tissue (Langer and Langer 1985). A periosteal releasing incision was then made with a #15 blade along the entire base of the recipient bed (Harris 1992) to facilitate advancement of the flap with coronal repositioning and to achieve partial root coverage. Debridement of exposed neck of the Brånemark implant surface was carried out with titanium curettes (Hu-Friedy) The advanced flap was stabilized with nine 6-0 sutures (Ethilon; Ethicon, Johnson & Johnson, New Brunswick, DE, USA) (Fig 8), with analgesics prescribed for pain control. The patient was then instructed to use chlorhexidine digluconate mouthwash for seven days, with suture removal planned for this time. An acrylic denture served as interim replacement for crown 21, with the denture adjusted to eliminate any pressure on the augmented area.

The grafted site was left to heal for twelve weeks, when the site was reentered in a second surgical procedure (Figs 9a-b). A significant increase in the thickness of the keratinized attached mucosal tissue was seen at this time, with an increase in the proximal tissue thickness in both the mesial and distal regions observed at the fixture-level impression appointment (Figs 10a-b).

N. MacBeth, N. Donos

Probing pocket depths recorded at this time (Fig 11) indicated an increase in the height of the gingival collar of implant 21 to 4 mm, with tissue recession at site 22 reduced by 2 to 3 mm. The pocketing in the maxillary right quadrant was also reduced, with the patient's bleeding and plaque scores maintained at less than 3%.

The replacement prosthetic crown was manufactured with an increased emergence profile to encourage proliferation of the interproximal papilla tissue and to reduce the interproximal spacing in this region. The new custom abutment junction was set at the established gingival level to ensure that the crown/abutment junction was accessible for cleaning (Figs 12a-b).

REC	132	101	222	122	221	121	000		222	133	222	222	233	200	000
PPD (P)	333	333	223	222	222	222	222	444	222	222	222	222	333	334	334
PPD (B)	333	222	222	222	222	223	222	434	222	222	322	223	333	433	334
Tooth position	17	16	15	14	13	12	11	21	22	23	24	25	26	27	28
Tooth position	47	46	45	44	43	42	41	31	32	33	34	35	36	37	38
PPD (B)	333	322	222	222	322	222	222	222	222	222	222	323	233	333	333
PPD (L)	333	323	222	222	222	222	222	222	222	222	223	322	333	334	433
REC	001	000	121	122	221	000	021	000	021	232	232	222	110	000	000

Fig 11　Probing pocket depths taken prior to exposure of the implant.

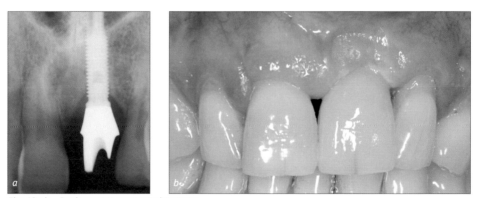

Figs 12a-b　Replacement crown at placement.

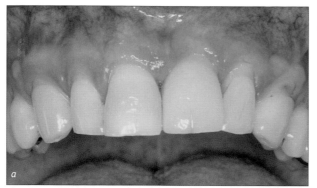
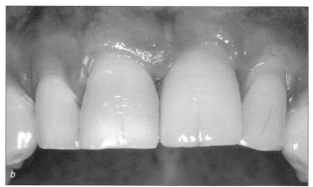

Figs 13a-c   Clinical situation two years after the placement of the new crown.

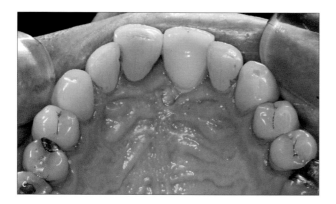

	17	16	15	14	13	12	11	21	22	23	24	25	26	27	28
REC	132	101	222	122	221	121	000	011	222	133	222	222	233	200	
PPD (P)	333	333	223	222	222	222	222	444	222	222	222	222	333	334	334
PPD (B)	333	222	222	222	222	223	222	434	222	222	322	223	333	433	334
Tooth position	17	16	15	14	13	12	11	21	22	23	24	25	26	27	28
Tooth position	47	46	45	44	43	42	41	31	32	33	34	35	36	37	38
PPD (B)	333	322	222	222	322	222	222	222	222	222	222	323	233	333	333
PPD (L)	333	323	222	222	222	222	222	222	222	222	223	322	333	334	433
REC	001	000	121	122	221	000	021	000	021	232	232	222	110	000	000

Fig 14   Full-mouth pocket chart two years after the placement of the prosthetic restoration.

A review of the prosthetic structure two years after placement indicated minimal change in the gingival collar position, with the partial tissue coverage gained following the grafting procedure still stable (Thoma and coworkers 2014) (Figs 13a-c).

Discussion

Successful implant outcomes are underpinned by positioning the implant at the optimal vertical and horizontal position within the alveolar bone, encouraging the development of a healthy peri-implant soft-tissue collar (Garber 1996) and reducing the risks of peri-implant mucosal complications (Mezzomo and coworkers 2011; de Lange 1994; Bartee 2005).

The characteristics of the peri-implant mucosa collar is an important feature in the success of dental implants (Tinti and Parma-Benfenati, 2012). The gingival morphology of the keratinized tissue (Abrahamsson and coworkers 1999) and the volume of the peri-implant mucosa (Abrahamsson and coworkers 1999; Puisys and Linkevicius 2015) have been reported as influencing marginal bone loss during the formation of the peri-implant tissues and affecting the long-term stability of the mucosal margin (Zarb and Schmitt 1990; Thoma and coworkers 2018b).

A wider keratinized tissue margin is potentially advantageous (Zarb and Schmitt 1990), as the margin has been suggested to be helpful in resisting mucosal inflammation (Bassetti and coworkers 2017), increasing the volume of extracellular matrix (Cardaropoli and coworkers 2006; Giannobile and coworkers 2018), and enhancing the body's regenerative response (Nauta and coworkers 2011; Chappuis and coworkers 2017).

When a peri-implant mucosal margin of less that 3 mm was found in a patient with a thin gingival phenotype, a greater risk of additional alveolar bone and soft-tissue loss was observed (Thoma and coworkers 2014; Thoma and coworkers 2018b). This finding suggests that emphasis should be given to the maintenance and retention of the keratinized tissue, as well as implant placement with a combined connective-tissue graft to compensate for gingival remodeling during healing (Thoma and coworkers 2014; Thoma and coworkers 2018) or surgical augmentation of the peri-implant mucosal margin if recession occurs (Bassetti and coworkers; Jepsen and coworkers 2015).

Various augmentation techniques are available to the clinician and include the use of autologous tissue free gingival grafts (Simons and coworkers 1993), connective-tissue grafts (Wiesner and coworkers 2010), xenografts (Sanz and coworkers 2009), or allografts. Although opinions on the optimal soft-tissue augmentation approach differ, the use of autologous connective-tissue grafts have been found to be the most effective at increasing the mucosal thickness and the size of the keratinized margin (Thoma and coworkers 2014; Giannobile and coworkers 2018; Bassetti and coworkers 2017).

After healing, connective-tissue graft sites were also observed to suffer from significantly less marginal bone loss, no significant changes in bleeding on probing, probing depths, or plaque scores (Lin and coworkers 2013; Gobbato and coworkers 2013). Augmented sites also had higher esthetic scores and better esthetic outcomes (Thoma and coworkers 2014), with only a small risk of post healing recession and site morbidity (Bassetti and coworkers 2017; Giannobile and coworkers 2018)

The functional and esthetic improvements achieved in this case demonstrates that a connective-tissue graft in combination with a coronally positioned graft is an effective method of treating cases with peri-implant mucositis and an associated abutment-level sinus abscess.

6.10   Covering a Soft-Tissue Dehiscence at a Mandibular Incisor

M. Roccuzzo

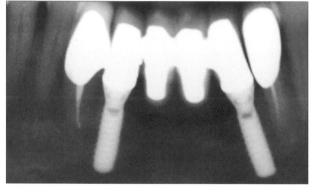

Fig 1   Post-treatment panoramic radiograph showing implants 32 and 42 supporting a four-unit bridge.

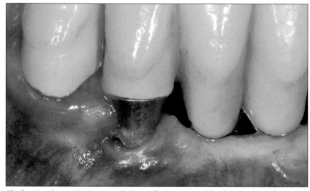

Fig 2   Implant 42. Accumulation of plaque on the implant surface and peri-implant mucositis.

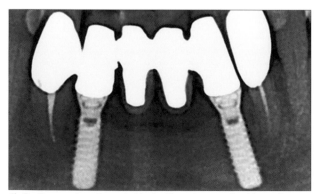

Fig 3   Panoramic radiograph. No significant interproximal bone change.

A 70-year-old woman was referred in September 2003 for implant placement to replace the four lower incisors. After initial periodontal preparation and the assurance of good oral-hygiene motivation and compliance, with a full-mouth plaque score (FMPS) of less than 25% and a full-mouth bleeding score (FMBS) of less than 25%, two implants (Tissue Level S RN, diameter 3.3 mm, length 12 mm; Institut Straumann AG, Basel, Switzerland) were placed at sites 32 and 42 to support a four-unit bridge. The surgical and restorative procedures were uneventful with no complications. After cementation of the bridge, a radiograph was taken (Fig 1). Baseline peri-implant probing confirmed the absence of pockets deeper than 4 mm.

The patient was placed on an individually tailored supportive periodontal/peri-implant therapy program (SPT), including continuous evaluation of the risk of biological complications. She was recalled at various intervals for motivation, reinstruction in oral hygiene procedures, and supragingival instrumentation as needed.

In November 2012, the patient came to the office to complain of discomfort and tenderness in the right mandibular region, which had been present for several weeks. Clinical examination revealed peri-implant soft-tissue inflammation at site 42. An accumulation of soft deposits on the coronal portion of implant 42 could be seen with the naked eye (Fig 2). The panoramic radiograph (Fig 3) displayed no significant proximal bone loss around either of the implants. A diagnosis of peri-implant mucositis associated with a soft-tissue dehiscence was made.

Non-surgical therapy should always be performed before any surgical intervention, as this gives time for the clinician to evaluate the healing response of the tissues, as well as the patient's ability to perform effective oral hygiene (Renvert and Polyzois 2015). The initial treatment consisted in careful debridement and cleaning of the area using titanium curettes and an ultrasonic device with a PTFE-coated tip to reduce the risk of damage to the implant surface. The implant was also polished with a rubber cup and polishing paste. Further ultrasonic debridement of calculus deposits in the remainder of the oral cavity was completed.

Six weeks later, in January 2013, the patient returned for a review. The clinical picture demonstrated a significant improvement of the soft-tissue conditions with a reduction in the accumulation of plaque deposits in the region (Fig 4).

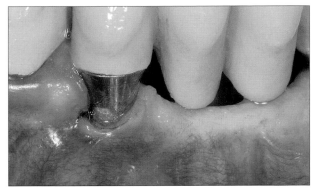

Fig 4   After the non-surgical initial treatment, the reduction of the soft-tissue inflammation was evident.

Although the initial non-surgical treatment reduced the inflammation of the peri-implant mucosa inflammation, a portion of the rough surface of the dental implant was still visible. There is sufficient evidence indicating that rough implant surfaces, left exposed to bacterial contamination, may constitute an additional risk factor for further biological complications (Louropoulou and coworkers 2012; Bermejo and coworkers 2019). Nevertheless, there is a lack of evidence regarding the optimal treatment for such situations.

Three therapeutic options were discussed with the patient including their relative advantages and disadvantages:

- The first was to simply smoothen the surface of the portion of implant exposed to the oral cavity by means of different burs to facilitate effective plaque removal by the patient. This option would be minimally invasive, but it would not create an effective protecting barrier around the implant.
- The second was to attempt guided bone regeneration around the implant using a bone graft and membrane to try to restore the original situation. A GBR procedure is always a sensitive surgical intervention, dependent on optimal bone graft stabilization and primary wound closure. In the present scenario, this would be even more difficult and would require the removal of the bridge.
- The third option was to attempt to correct the dehiscence by means of a connective-tissue graft. Following a discussion with the patient about the advantages and disadvantages of each treatment modality, it was decided that the third option would be preferable.

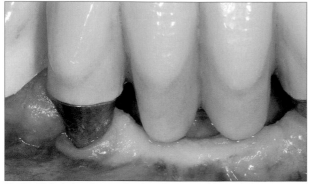

Fig 5   Clinical situation on the day of surgery with good plaque control and no signs of inflammation.

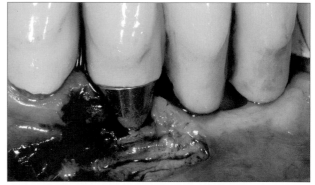

Fig 6   Split-thickness trapezoidal flap elevated on the buccal side of the implant. Facial aspects of the anatomical papillae de-epithelized to create connective-tissue beds for the coronally advanced flap.

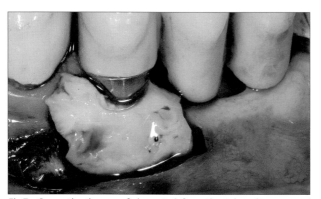

Fig 7   Connective-tissue graft harvested from the tuberosity area and trimmed to a U-shape, adapted to the collar of the implant.

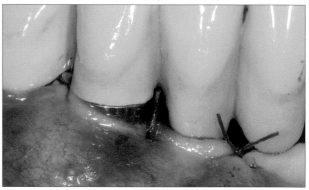

Fig 8   Graft sutured to the recipient bed and covered by a coronally advanced flap with minimal tension.

On the day of surgery, the patient presented with good plaque control and no significant signs of bleeding, allowing the treatment to be performed under ideal conditions (Fig 5).

An intracrevicular incision was made on the buccal aspect of the affected implant, and a split-thickness trapezoidal buccal flap was elevated. The facial portion of the interdental papillae were de-epithelized to expose connective-tissue beds for the adaptation of the coronally advanced flap. Several procedures have been employed and tested for the decontamination of implant surfaces, but so far there has been no evidence that one of them is superior (Schwarz and coworkers 2011; Subramani and Wismeijer 2012). In this case, the implant surface was dried with gauze and 24% ethylenediaminetetraacetic acid (EDTA) (Prefgel; Institut Straumann AG) applied to all exposed threads, followed by application of a 1% chlorhexidine gel (Corsodyl dental gel; GlaxoSmithKline, Baranzate, Italy), each for two minutes. The surface was rinsed thoroughly with sterile saline solution (Fig 6).

A thick connective-tissue graft was excised from the tuberosity area, de-epithelialized with a blade, and trimmed to a U-shape with a mucotome for optimal adaptation to the collar of the implant, which was 4.1 mm in diameter. The thickness of the mucosal graft was approximately 2 mm (Fig 7).

The prepared connective-tissue graft was sutured to the recipient bed, and the buccal flap was sutured coronally to cover the graft with minimal tension. Immediately after surgery, the patient was advised to apply an ice pack over the treated area, recommending that this continue for at least four hours. She was also instructed to avoid tooth brushing and trauma to the surgical site for three weeks, and to use a 0.2% chlorhexidine digluconate rinse for one minute three times a day during the same period (Fig 8).

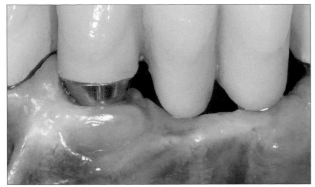

Fig 9 *Clinical situation at the follow-up examination at one year.*

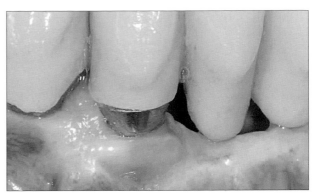

Fig 10 *Follow-up examination at two years.*

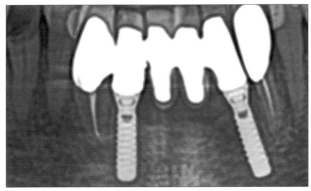

Fig 11 *Panoramic radiograph at three years confirming the maintenance of stable proximal bone levels.*

The patient was seen again after one week to monitor healing and after two weeks for removal of the sutures. After that, she was seen weekly for the first four weeks and then every three months for the first year. Motivation, reinforcement of oral hygiene, and instrumentation was performed as needed. The one-year clinical photograph revealed complete soft-tissue coverage of the rough surface of the implant (Fig 9).

After the first year, the patient was placed on an individualized SPT program, which included continuous evaluation of the occurrence and the risk of biological complications (Roccuzzo and coworkers 2014a) (Figs 10 and 11).

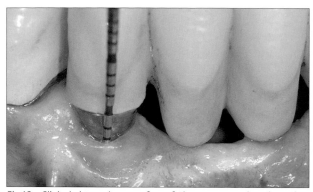

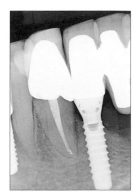

Fig 13   Periapical   radiograph   at six years (fifteen years after implant placement).

Fig 12   Clinical picture six years after soft-tissue surgery, when the patient was 85 years old. Increased thickness of the soft tissues and no peri-implant bleeding on probing.

The last clinical picture, taken in November 2018 when the patient was 85 years old—6 years after the connective-tissue graft—revealed stable soft-tissue contours and no signs of inflammation or significant recession (Fig 12). The radiograph demonstrated the stability of the interproximal bone, fifteen years after implant placement (Fig 13). With this patient's history in mind, it is advisable to place implants with a long-term vision, so that maintenance is easy both for the patient and the dentist.

To reduce the risk of exposure of the implant surface, it is imperative to place the implants such that they are surrounded by an adequate thickness of bone. Furthermore, to avoid bacterial contamination that could jeopardize the long-term success of implants, the early establishment of a long-standing effective soft-tissue barrier, capable of biologically protecting the peri-implant structures, is mandatory (Rompen and coworkers 2006). If, for any reason. this soft-tissue seal were broken or damaged, it could be restored in a manner similar to the one presented in this case. Further long-term controlled studies are necessary to assess the most effective surgical techniques for soft-tissue reconstruction.

Acknowledgments

Laboratory procedures
Francesco Cataldi, Master Dental Technician – Torino, Italy

Oral hygiene procedures
Silvia Gherlone, Registered Dental Hygienist – Torino, Italy

6.11 Soft-Tissue Augmentation Using a Porcine-Derived Collagen Matrix to Correct a Labial Soft-Tissue Defect Following Extraction of a Maxillary Incisor

S. Shahdad

Soft-tissue defects are often encountered prior to implant placement and may result in deficient attached keratinized mucosa, which unless corrected will yield less than ideal esthetic outcomes. The presence of keratinized mucosa has been proposed as one of the prognostic factors for the survival of dental implants (Adell and coworkers 1986) with reported greater reductions in gingival and plaque indices after increasing the width of keratinized mucosa by soft-tissue augmentation (Giannobile and coworkers 2018; Thoma and coworkers 2018). A lack of keratinized mucosa around implants makes the peri-implant mucosa more susceptible to inflammation, causing bone loss in ligature-induced animal studies (Warrer and coworkers 1995). Human studies have demonstrated similar results (Chung and coworkers 2006), including increased recession (Artzi and coworkers 2006); however, no impact on implant survival was demonstrated (Chung and coworkers 2006).

Conventionally, free gingival grafts (Sullivan and Atkins 1969) or subepithelial connective-tissue grafts (Edel 1974) have been used to repair soft-tissue deficiencies. Harvesting autologous soft tissue has inherent disadvantages, including the need for a remote surgical site for harvesting, often with a limited amount of donor tissue available for grafting. Healed free gingival grafts may present a mismatch in shade and texture with the adjacent tissues, whereas connective-tissue grafts offer better esthetics and shade matching (Roccuzzo and coworkers 2002; Orsini and coworkers 2004). However, both techniques are associated with significant patient morbidity due to the need for a second surgical site in the palate.

To reduce patient morbidity, acellular dermal allografts have been used as a substitute for autologous tissue in soft-tissue augmentation for increasing the width of the attached gingiva/mucosa around teeth or implants and as a socket seal in ridge preservation (Wei and coworkers 2002; Harris 2003; Park 2006; Yan and coworkers 2006; Imberman 2007).

Another option is the use of porcine-derived collagen membranes, which are an accepted treatment modality in guided bone regeneration (GBR) (Mitchell 1986; Hämmerle and Jung 2003; Hämmerle and coworkers 2002, Wallace and Froun 2003, Rastogi and coworkers 2009). Different collagen barrier membranes and matrices have been used to provide soft-tissue coverage over extraction sites and bone grafts in ridge preservation (Jung and coworkers 2004).

Recently, a two-layer, porcine-derived collagen matrix (CMX) (Mucograft; Geistlich Pharma, Wolhusen, Switzerland) has been investigated for the treatment of dehiscence defects around teeth (McGuire and Schreyer 2010) and for augmenting keratinized tissue around teeth and implant-supported fixed restorations (Sanz and coworkers 2009; Herford and coworkers 2010; Froum and coworkers 2015). A similar increase in the amount of keratinized tissue was demonstrated when the xenogeneic soft-tissue substitute was compared with autologous connective-tissue grafts (CTG) (Sanz and coworkers 2009).

The matrix is of type I and type III collagen and is thicker than conventional collagen membranes. During healing, the newly formed soft tissue (gingiva/mucosa) at the matrix periphery grows through it rather than underneath it, as it is replacing it (Herford and coworkers 2010). Furthermore, the vascular flow changes after the application of CMX when used for root coverage did not present significant differences compared to the use of CTG (Tatarakis and coworkers 2018).

There have been no published reports for the application of CMX in repairing soft-tissue defects prior to implant placement. In the present clinical case, CMX was used to repair a soft-tissue defect six weeks begore implant placement with simultaneous GBR.

Case report

A 45-year-old healthy, non-smoking man presented with an epithelialized soft-tissue tunnel defect (Fig 1a-c). The patient exercised good oral hygiene, with a full-mouth bleeding score (FMBS) under 20%. Full-mouth probing did not reveal any pockets deeper than 3 to 4 mm.

Tooth 11 had been extracted six weeks previously, and it was planned to replace it with an implant using simultaneous GBR. Some interdental bone loss with less than 1 mm of gingival recession was noted at teeth 12 and 21 (Miller class 3 recession).

The soft-tissue defect was considered a high risk for implant placement. The superficial bridge of tissue was excised and the underlying tissue de-epithelialized to create a fresh bleeding bed for the graft. A CMX matrix was inserted into the pouch and stabilized with single interrupted 6-0 monofilament nylon sutures (Seralon; Serag-Wiessner, Naila, Germany) (Fig 2a-c).

After one week, healing with minimal surface sloughing was evident. The graft continued to mature over six weeks (Fig 3a-b), when implant surgery was performed. A multi-wall bone defect including communication with the nasopalatine canal was noted, with proximal bone loss on the adjacent teeth (Fig 4a-b).

An implant (Tissue Level SLActive SP RN, diameter 3.3 mm, length 10 mm ; Institut Straumann AG, Basel Switzerland) was placed in an ideal three-dimensional position for a screw-retained restoration resulting in an 8-mm labial and mesial dehiscence of the roughened surface of the implant. Simultaneous GBR was carried out. Autologous bone shavings were collected from the adjacent area and placed over the implant, followed by blood-soaked deproteinized bovine bone substitute (BioOss; Geistlich Pharma), which was covered by a bi-layer porcine-derived collagen barrier membrane (BioGide, Geistlich Pharma). In order to minimize post-surgical recession, the upper right lateral incisor and the upper left central incisor were treated with enamel matrix derivative (Emdogain; Institut Straumann AG) (Fig 5a-f). The wound was closed with coronally repositioned flaps and single interrupted 5-0 monofilament nylon sutures (Seralon; Serag-Wiessner).

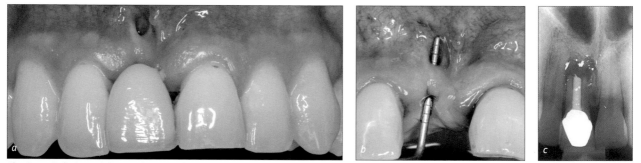

Figs 1a-c   Soft tissue defect at the apex of previously extracted tooth 11 (a). Epithelialized soft-tissue tunnel defect at the implant site (b). Periapical baseline radiograph (c).

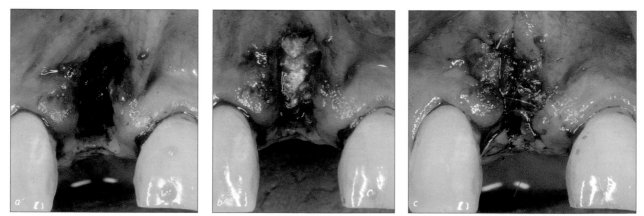

Figs 2a-c   Superficial bridge of epithelialized tissue excised and the underlying tissue de-epithelialized (a). Collagen matrix (Mucograft) adapted and placed into a pouch underneath the flap edges (b). Single interrupted sutures to stabilize the matrix without complete coverage of the graft (c).

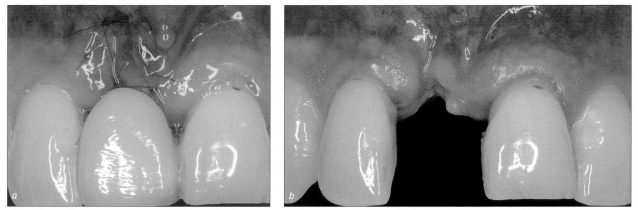

Figs 3a-b   Healing progress at one week (a). Graft healing and maturation at six weeks, immediately prior to implant surgery (b).

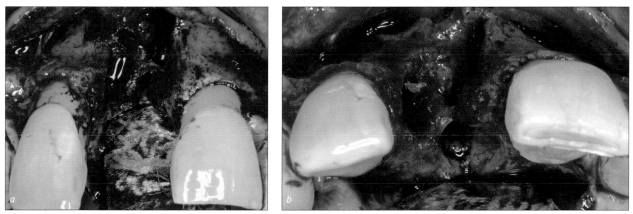

Figs 4a-b   Severity of the bone defect, including communication with nasopalatine canal and loss of interdental bone on the adjacent teeth.

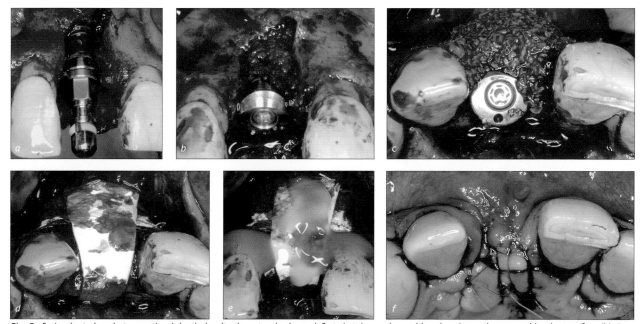

Figs 5a-f   Implant placed at an optimal depth despite the extensive bone defect. Autologous bone chips placed over the exposed implant surface (b). Buccal and palatal bone regenerated using deproteinized bovine bone substitute (c). A double layer of porcine collagen membrane placed over the particulate bone substitute (d). Enamel matrix derivate applied to the adjacent root surface and the grafting site (e). Tension-free primary closure (f).

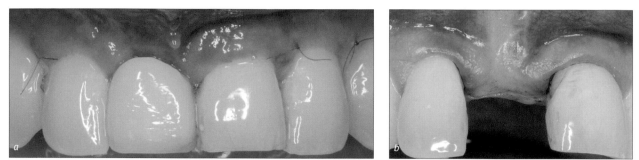

Figs 6a-b Healing progress one week after the implantation (a). Healing at eight weeks, immediately prior to exposure of the implant(b). Loss of interdental papillae on the proximal surfaces of the adjacent teeth.

The sutures were removed after a week and the implant was exposed after eight weeks (Fig 6a-b), at which time papilla reconstruction was attempted with two laterally rotating pedicle flaps (Fig 7a-c).

A laboratory-made provisional crown was used to manipulate the soft tissues to optimize the pink esthetics (Fig 7d). The incisal wear of tooth 21 was corrected by a direct composite-resin restoration. The patient followed a maintenance protocol with biannual review and hygienist appointments.

After three years, a 4-mm band of keratinized peri-implant mucosa and a mucogingival line with optimal shade and texture was noted (Fig 8). A deficiency of the mesial and distal papillae remained, which is consistent with the preoperative interdental bone loss on the adjacent teeth. The three-year follow-up radiograph demonstrated stable bone levels. The CBCT shows 4.7 mm of labial bone at the thickest point and 2.7 mm at the SLActive/smooth surface junction. Bone is present coronal to this junction (Fig 9a-b).

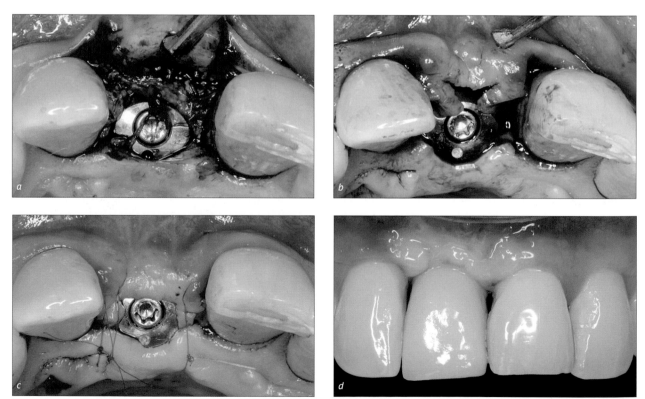

Figs 7a-d Minimal crestal flap elevation showing the extent of bone regeneration on the buccal aspect (a). Papilla reconstruction attempted with laterally repositioned pedicle flaps (b). Adaptation of pedicled papillae with simple interrupted sutures (c). Provisional restoration at delivery (d).

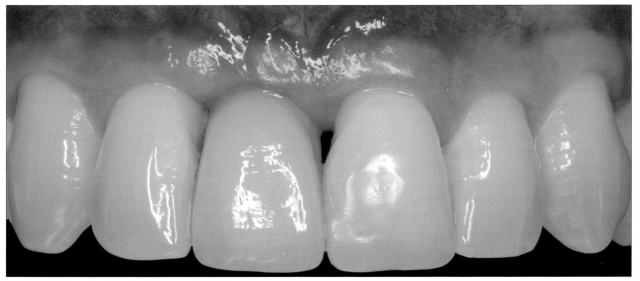

Fig 8   Definitive restoration after three years in function.

Discussion

This clinical case demonstrates soft-tissue repair in a post-extraction healed site using a porcine collagen matrix. The anticipated quantitative and qualitative outcomes to match the adjacent areas were achieved. Based on the Pink Esthetic Score index (Fürhauser and coworkers 2005), a total score of 12/14 was achieved, with deficiencies noted at the mesial and distal papillae. This is the first such reported case illustrating soft-tissue defect repair with a porcine collagen matrix prior to implantation. However, the level of supporting evidence is weak, and there is a need for randomized controlled clinical trials to establish higher-level evidence.

After one week, healing with surface sloughing was evident, and although the matrix was left uncovered, the area was completely epithelialized in two weeks. The soft-tissue healing and repair at six weeks the operative site barely discernable from the adjacent areas. The shade match and regeneration of keratinized tissue was adequate to facilitate restoration with an implant.

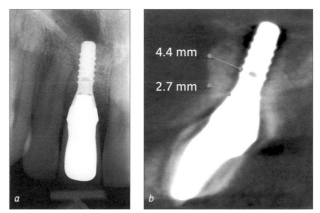

Figs 9a-b   Periapical radiograph at three years (a). CBCT scan of the implant showing regeneration of labial bone at three years (b).

Volume 12 of the ITI Treatment Guide series has clearly demonstrated that for dental implants:

- Osseointegration is simple.
- Soft-tissue integration is difficult.
- Long-term maintenance is complicated.

While osseointegration can be predictably achieved in most circumstances, soft-tissue integration around dental implants is often clinically challenging. Furthermore, the long-term maintenance of peri-implant health may be complicated due to issues related to the condition of the soft tissue present in the area.

In implant dentistry, the attention of clinicians and researchers has primarily been focused on the bone-to-implant interface, based on the observation that implant placement is a safe and predictable procedure. Nevertheless, the possibility of biological complications can never be excluded, even after appropriate diagnosis and meticulous treatment planning. The vast majority of these complications originate within the peri-implant marginal soft tissue. Consequently, there is a need for dental practitioners to gain additional knowledge and to focus more on the status of this soft tissue.

Clinicians placing dental implants need to understand the difficulties that arise from biological complications and should make every effort to avoid them, by creating conditions that render self-performed oral hygiene measures as easy as possible for the patient. The long-term success of a dental implant can be associated with both the standard of plaque control and the health of the peri-implant mucosa. In this scenario, it is hard to analyze which of the two comes first: without proper plaque control, oral health cannot be achieved; on the other hand, it may be challenging for patients to perform proper oral hygiene if the soft tissue surrounding a dental implant is not healthy.

As a profession, we need to ensure that our patients receive adequate oral care and support following implant placement and restoration. The results of the most recent studies encourage continuous monitoring of peri-implant tissue conditions to prevent or detect early biological complications.

Dentists should pay attention to the status of the peri-implant soft tissue, particularly in situations where patients present with one or more of the following conditions:

- Soreness during oral hygiene procedures
- Thinning of the peri-implant mucosa subsequent to coronal flap advancement associated with bone regenerative procedures
- Suboptimal plaque control, that could be improved by optimizing the local anatomy
- Presence of peri-implant recession
- Shallow vestibule, particularly in the posterior mandible

In recent years, an increasing number of authors have started to focus on soft-tissue integration, i.e., the creation of an early and long-lasting effective barrier capable of biologically protecting the peri-implant structures.

The intention of this volume has been to provide clinicians with guidelines to establish healthy soft tissue around dental implants that may improve their long-term success, regardless of the initial clinical conditions.

The evaluation of the soft tissues should always be the starting point when planning implant placement, augmenting the soft and hard tissues around dental implants, or restoring these implants.

Clinical evidence for the significance of such monitoring is provided in several parts of this volume, as the key to success lies in the active and continuous cooperation and compliance of patients.

It is evident that in the future, peri-implant soft-tissue treatment will increasingly occupy the dental profession. Clinicians must understand that implant-supported restorations should be designed to offer easy access to oral hygiene, but soft-tissue manipulation is also necessary for a proper long-term self-maintenance of peri-implant tissue health.

It is the present authors' sincere wish and hope that this volume may remind all clinicians that periodontal therapy is always part of the overall comprehensive treatment associated with implant dentistry.

8   <u>References</u>

References have been listed in the order of (1) the first or only author's last name and (2) the year of publication. Identical short references are distinguished in the text by lowercase letters, which if used are given in parentheses at the end of the respective entry in this list of references.

Abrahamsson I, Berglundh T, Wennström J, Lindhe J. The peri-implant hard and soft tissues at different implant systems. A comparative study in the dog. Clin Oral Implants Res. **1996** Sep; 7(3): 212 – 219. doi: 10.1034/j.1600-0501.1996.070303.x.

Abrahamsson I, Berglundh T, Moon IS, Lindhe J. Peri-implant tissues at submerged and non-submerged titanium implants. J Clin Periodontol. **1999** Sep; 26(9): 600 – 607. doi: 10.1034/j.1600-051x.1999.260907.x.

Abrahamsson I, Zitzmann NU, Berglundh T, Wennerberg A, Lindhe J. Bone and soft tissue integration to titanium implants with different surface topography: an experimental study in the dog. Int J Oral Maxillofac Implants. **2001** May-Jun; 16(3): 323 – 332.

Abrahamsson I, Zitzmann NU, Berglundh T, Linder E, Wennerberg A, Lindhe J. The mucosal attachment to titanium implants with different surface characteristics: an experimental study in dogs. J Clin Periodontol. **2002** May; 29(5): 448 – 455. doi: 10.1034/j.1600-051x.2002.290510.x.

Adell R, Lekholm U, Rockler B, Brånemark PI, Lindhe J, Eriksson B, et al. Marginal tissue reactions at osseointegrated titanium fixtures (I). A 3-year longitudinal prospective study. Int J Oral Maxillofac Surg. **1986** Feb; 15(1): 39 – 52.

Adell R, Eriksson B, Lekholm U, Brånemark PI, Jemt T. Long-term follow-up study of osseointegrated implants in the treatment of totally edentulous jaws. Int J Oral Maxillofac Implants. **1990** Winter; 5(4): 347 – 359.

Adibrad M, Shahabuei M, Sahabi M. Significance of the width of keratinized mucosa on the health status of the supporting tissue around implants supporting overdentures. J Oral Implantol. **2009**; 35(5): 232 – 237. doi: 10.1563/AAID-JOI-D-09-00035.1.

Aglietta M, Iorio Siciliano V, Zwahlen M, Brägger U, Pjetursson BE, Lang NP, Salvi GE. A systematic review of the survival and complication rates of implant supported fixed dental prostheses with cantilever extension after an observation period of at least 5 years. Clin Oral Implants Res. **2009** May; 20(5): 441 – 451. doi: 10.1111/j.1600-0501.2009.01706.x.

Aglietta M, Iorio Siciliano V, Blasi A, Sculean A, Brägger U, Lang NP, Salvi GE. Clinical and radiographic changes at implants supporting single-unit crowns (SCs) and fixed dental prostheses (FDPs) with one cantilever extension. A retrospective study. Clin Oral Implants Res. **2012** May; 23(5): 550 – 555. doi: 10.1111/j.1600-0501.2011.02391.x.

Ainamo J, Löe H: Anatomic characteristics of gingiva. A clinical and microscopic study of the free and attached gingiva. J Periodontol. **1966**; 37(1): 5 – 13.

Akcalı A, Schneider D, Ünlü F, Bıcakcı N, Köse T, Hämmerle CH. Soft tissue augmentation of ridge defects in the maxillary anterior area using two different methods: a randomized controlled clinical trial. Clin Oral Implants Res. **2015** Jun; 26(6): 688 – 695. doi: 10.1111/clr.12368.

Akcalı A, Trullenque-Eriksson A, Sun C, Petrie A, Nibali L, Donos N. What is the effect of soft tissue thickness on crestal bone loss around dental implants? A systematic review. Clin Oral Implants Res. **2017** Sep; 28(9): 1046 – 1053. doi: 10.1111/clr.12916.

Albrektsson T, Brånemark PI, Hansso HA, Lindström J. Osseointegrated titanium implants. Requirements for ensuring a long-lasting, direct bone anchorage in man. Acta Orthop Scand. **1981**; 52: 155 – 170. doi: 10.3109/17453678108991776.

Allen AL. Use of the supraperiosteal envelope in soft tissue grafting for root coverage. I. Rationale and technique. Int J Periodontics Restorative Dent. **1994** Jun; 14(3): 216 – 227.

Allen EP, Miller PD Jr. Coronal positioning of existing gingiva: short term results in the treatment of shallow marginal tissue recession. J Periodontol. **1989** Jun; 60(6): 316 – 319. doi: 10.1902/jop.1989.60.6.316.

Allen EP. Subpapillary continuous sling suturing method for soft tissue grafting with the tunneling technique. Int J Periodontics Restorative Dent. **2010** Oct; 30(5): 479 – 485.

Amin PN, Bissada NF, Ricchetti PA, Silva APB, Demko CA. Tuberosity versus palatal donor sites for soft tissue grafting: A split-mouth clinical study. Quintessence Int. **2018**; 49(7): 589 – 598. doi: 10.3290/j.qi.a40510.

Anderson LE, Inglehart MR, El-Kholy K, Eber R, Wang HL. Implant associated soft tissue defects in the anterior maxilla: a randomized control trial comparing subepithelial connective tissue graft and acellular dermal matrix allograft. Implant Dent. **2014** Aug; 23(4): 416–425. doi: 10.1097/ID.0000000000000122.

Aroca S, Keglevitch T, Nikolidakis D, Gera I, Nagy K, Azzi R, Etienne D. Treatment of class III multiple gingival recessions: a randomized-clinical trial. J Clin Periodontol. **2010** Jan; 37(1): 88–97. doi: 10.1111/j.1600-051X.2009.01492.x.

Aroca S, Molnár B, Windisch P, Gera I, Salvi GE, Nikolidakis D, Sculean A. Treatment of multiple adjacent Miller class I and II gingival recessions with a modified coronally advanced tunnel (MCAT) technique and a collagen matrix or palatal connective tissue graft: a randomized, controlled clinical trial. J Clin Periodontol. **2013** Jul; 40(7): 713–720. doi: 10.1111/jcpe.12112.

Artzi Z, Carmeli G, Kozlovsky A. A distinguishable observation between survival and success rate outcome of hydroxyapatite-coated implants in 5–10 years in function. Clinical Oral Implants Research. **2006** Feb; 17(1): 85–93. doi: 10.1111/j.1600-0501.2005.01178.x.

Arvidson K, Fartash B, Hilliges M, Kondell PA. Histological characteristics of peri-implant mucosa around Brånemark and single-crystal sapphire implants. Clin Oral Implants Res. **1996** Mar; 7(1): 1–10. doi: 10.1034/j.1600-0501.1996.070101.x.

Assenza B, Scarano A, Petrone G, Iezzi G, Thams U, San Roman F, Piattelli A. Crestal bone remodeling in loaded and unloaded implants and the microgap: a histologic study. Implant Dent. **2003**; 12: 235–241. doi: 10.1097/01.id.0000074081.17978.7e.

Avila-Ortiz G, Chambrone L, Vignoletti F. Effect of alveolar ridge preservation interventions following tooth extraction: A systematic review and meta-analysis. J Clin Periodontol. **2019** Jun; 46 Suppl 21: 195–223. doi: 10.1111/jcpe.13057.

Azzi R, Etienne D, Davarpanah M. Subepithelial connective tissue graft in periodontal surgery. Indication for root coverage, esthetic purpose, and in treatment of osseous lesions: the sandwich technique. In: Gold S, Midda M, Mutlu S (eds). Recent advances in periodontology, Vol II. Amsterdam: Elsevier Science Publishers. **1991**; 251–256.

Azzi R, Etienne D. Recouvrement radiculaire et reconstruction papillaire par greffon conjonctif enfoui sous un lambeau vestibulaire tunnélisé et tracté coronairement. Journal de Parodontologie et d'Implantologie Orale. **1998** Feb; 17(1): 71–77.

Barone R, Clauser C, Prato GP. Localized soft tissue ridge augmentation at phase 2 implant surgery: a case report. Int J Periodontics Restorative Dent. **1999** Apr; 19(2): 141–145.

Bartee B. Esthetic considerations in implant dentistry. Tex Dent J. **2005** Apr; 122(4): 318–331.

Bartold PM, Walsh LJ, Narayanan AS: Molecular and cell biology of the gingiva. Periodontol 2000. **2000** Oct; 24: 28–55. doi: 10.1034/j.1600-0757.2000.2240103.x.

Başeğmez C, Ersanlı S, Demirel K, Bölükbaşı N, Yalçın S. The comparison of two techniques to increase the amount of peri-implant attached mucosa: free gingival grafts versus vestibuloplasty. One-year results from a randomised controlled trial. Eur J Oral Implantol. **2012** Summer; 5(2): 139–145.

Başeğmez C, Karabuda ZC, Demirel K, Yalçın S. The comparison of acellular dermal matrix allografts with free gingival grafts in the augmentation of peri-implant attached mucosa: a randomised controlled trial. Eur J Oral Implantol. **2013** Summer; 6(2): 145–152.

Bassetti RG, Stähli A, Bassetti MA, Sculean A. Soft tissue augmentation around osseointegrated and uncovered dental implants: a systematic review. Clin Oral Investig. **2017** Jan; 21(1): 53–70. doi: 10.1007/s00784-016-2007-9.

Belser U, Buser D, Higginbottom F. Consensus statements and recommended clinical procedures regarding esthetics in implant dentistry. Int J Oral Maxillofac Implants. **2004**; 19 Suppl: 73–74.

Bengazi F, Wennström JL, Lekholm U. Recession of the soft tissue margin at oral implants. A 2-year longitudinal prospective study. Clin Oral Implants Res. **1996** Dec; 7(4): 303–310. doi: 10.1034/j.1600-0501.1996.070401.x.

Bengazi F, Lang N, Caroprese M, Urbizo Velez J, Favero V, Botticelli D. Dimensional changes in soft tissues around dental implants following free gingival grafting: an experimental study in dogs. Clin Oral Implants Res. **2015** Feb; 26(2): 176–183. doi: 10.1111/clr.12280.

Benic GI, Hämmerle CH. Horizontal bone augmentation by means of guided bone regeneration. Periodontology 2000. **2014** Oct; 66(1): 13 – 40. doi: 10.1111/prd.12039.

Berglundh T, Lindhe J, Ericsson I, Marinello CP, Liljenberg B, Thomsen P. The soft tissue barrier at implants and teeth. Clin Oral Implants Res. **1991** Apr – Jun; 2(2) :81 – 90. doi: 10.1034/j.1600-0501.1991.020206.x.

Berglundh T, Lindhe J. Dimension of the periimplant mucosa. Biological width revisited. J Clin Periodontol. **1996** Oct; 23(10): 971 – 973. doi: 10.1111/j.1600-051x.1996.tb00520.x.

Berglundh T, Abrahamsson I, Welander M, Lang NP, Lindhe J. Morphogenesis of the peri-implant mucosa: an experimental study in dogs. Clin Oral Implants Res. **2007** Feb; 18(1): 1 – 8. doi: 10.1111/j.1600-0501.2006.01380.x.

Berglundh T, Zitzmann NU, Donati M. Are peri-implantitis lesions different from periodontitis lesions? J Clin Periodontol. **2011** Mar; 38 Suppl 11: 188 – 202. doi: 10.1111/j.1600-051X.2010.01672.x.

Berglundh T, Armitage G, Araújo MG, Avila-Ortiz G, Blanco J, Camargo PM, Chen S, Cochran D, Derks J, Figuero E, Hämmerle CHF, Heitz-Mayfield LJA, Huynh-Ba G, Iacono V, Koo KT, Lambert F, McCauley L, Quirynen M, Renvert S, Salvi GE, Schwarz F, Tarnow D, Tomasi C, Wang HL, Zitzmann N. Peri-implant diseases and conditions: Consensus report of workgroup 4 of the 2017 World Workshop on the Classification of Periodontal and Peri-Implant Diseases and Conditions. J Periodontol. **2018** Jun; 89 Suppl 1: S313 – S318. doi: 10.1002/JPER.17-0739.

Bermejo P, Sánchez MC, Llama-Palacios A, Figuero E, Herrera D, Sanz Alonso M. Biofilm formation on dental implants with different surface micro-topography: An in vitro study. Clin Oral Implants Res. **2019** Aug; 30(8): 725 – 734. doi: 10.1111/clr.13455.

Bonino F, Steffensen B, Natto Z, Hur Y, Holtzman LP, Weber HP. Prospective study of the impact of peri-implant soft tissue properties on patient-reported and clinically assessed outcomes. J Periodontol. 2018; 89(9): 1025 – 1032. doi: 10.1002/JPER.18-0031.

Block MS, Gardiner D, Kent JN, Misiek DJ, Finger IM, Guerra L. Hydroxyapatite-coated cylindrical implants in the posterior mandible: 10-year observations. Int J Oral Maxillofac Implants. **1996** Sep – Oct; 11(5): 626 – 633.

Bosshardt DD, Lang NP: The junctional epithelium: from health to disease. J Dent Res. **2005** Jan; 84(1): 9 – 20. doi: 10.1177/154405910508400102.

Bouri A Jr, Bissada N, Al-Zahrani MS, Faddoul F, Nouneh I. Width of keratinized gingiva and the health status of the supporting tissues around dental implants. Int J Oral Maxillofac Implants. **2008** Mar – Apr; 23(2): 323 – 326.

Boynueğri D, Nemli SK, Kasko YA. Significance of keratinized mucosa around dental implants: a prospective comparative study. Clin Oral Implants Res. **2013** Aug; 24(8): 928 – 933. doi: 10.1111/j.1600-0501.2012.02475.x.

Brito C, Tenenbaum HC, Wong BK, Schmitt C, Nogueira-Filho G. Is keratinized mucosa indispensable to maintain peri-implant health? A systematic review of the literature. J Biomed Mater Res B Appl Biomater. **2014** Apr; 102(3): 643 – 650. doi: 10.1002/jbm.b.33042.

Bruno JF. Connective tissue graft technique assuring wide root coverage. nt J Periodontics Restorative Dent. **1994** Apr; 14(2): 126 – 137.

Buchi DL, Sailer I, Fehmer V, Hämmerle CH, Thoma DS. All-ceramic single-tooth implant reconstructions using modified zirconia abutments: a prospective randomized controlled clinical trial of the effect of pink veneering ceramic on the esthetic outcomes. Int J Periodontics Restorative Dent. **2014** Jan – Feb; 34(1): 29 – 37. doi: 10.11607/prd.1870.

Burkhardt R, Andreoni C, Marinello CP. Psychological and social effects of implant supported reconstructions. ACTA Med Denti Helv. **2000**; 5: 1 – 8.

Burkhardt R, Joss A, Lang NP. Soft tissue dehiscence coverage around endosseous implants: a prospective cohort study. Clin Oral Implant Res. **2008** May; 19(5): 451 – 457. doi: 10.1111/j.1600-0501.2007.01497.x.

Buser D, Weber HP, Donath K, Fiorellini JP, Paquette DW, Williams RC. Soft tissue reactions to non-submerged unloaded titanium implants in beagle dogs. J Periodontol. **1992** Mar; 63(3): 225 – 235. doi: 10.1902/jop.1992.63.3.225.

Buser D, Martin W, Belser UC. Optimizing esthetics for implant restorations in the anterior maxilla: anatomic and surgical considerations. Int J Oral Maxillofac Implants. **2004**; 19 Suppl: 43 – 61.

Buser D, Chen ST, Weber HP, Belser UC. Early implant placement following single-tooth extraction in the esthetic zone: biologic rationale and surgical procedures. Int J Periodontics Restorative Dent. **2008** Oct; 28(5): 441–451.

Buser D, Halbritter S, Hart C, Bornstein MM, Grütter L, Chappuis V, Belser UC. Early implant placement with simultaneous guided bone regeneration following single-tooth extraction in the esthetic zone: 12-month results of a prospective study with 20 consecutive patients. J Periodontol. **2009** Jan; 80(1): 152–162. doi: 10.1902/jop.2009.080360.

Buser D, Janner SF, Wittneben JG, Brägger U, Ramseier CA, Salvi GE. 10-year survival and success rates of 511 titanium implants with a sandblasted and acid-etched surface: a retrospective study in 303 partially edentulous patients. Clin Implant Dent Relat Res. **2012** Dec; 14(6): 839–851. doi: 10.1111/j.1708-8208.2012.00456.x.

Büyüközdemir Aşkın S, Berker E, Akıncıbay H, Uysal S, Erman B, Tezcan İ, Karabulut E. Necessity of keratinized tissues for dental implants: a clinical, immunological, and radiographic study. Clin Implant Dent Relat Res. **2015** Feb; 17(1): 1–12. doi: 10.1111/cid.12079.

Cairo F, Pagliaro U, Nieri M. Soft tissue management at implant sites. J Clin Periodontol. **2008** Sep; 35(8 Suppl): 163–167. doi: 10.1111/j.1600-051X.2008.01266.x.

Cairo F, Nieri M, Cincinelli S, Mervelt J, Pagliaro U. The interproximal clinical attachment level to classify gingival recessions and predict root coverage outcomes: an explorative and reliability study. J Clin Periodontol. **2011** Jul; 38(7): 661–666. doi: 10.1111/j.1600-051X.2011.01732.x.

Cairo F, Nieri M, Pagliaro U. Efficacy of periodontal plastic surgery procedures in the treatment of localized facial gingival recessions. A systematic review. J Clin Periodontol. **2014** Apr; 41 Suppl 15: S44–S62. doi: 10.1111/jcpe.12182.

Cairo F, Barbato L, Tonelli P, Batalocco G, Pagavino G, Nieri M. Xenogeneic collagen matrix versus connective tissue graft for buccal soft tissue augmentation at implant site. A randomized, controlled clinical trial. J Clin Periodontol. **2017** Jul; 44(7): 769–776. doi: 10.1111/jcpe.12750.

Caplanis N, Romanos G, Rosens P, Bickert G, Sharma A, Lozada J. Teeth versus implants: mucogingival considerations and management of soft tissue complications. J Calif Dent Assoc. **2014** Dec; 42(12): 841–858.

Cardaropoli G, Lekholm U, Wennström JL. Tissue alterations at implant-supported single-tooth replacements: a 1-year prospective clinical study. Clin Oral Implants Res. **2006** Apr; 17(2): 165–171. doi: 10.1111/j.1600-0501.2005.01210.x.

Caton JG, Armitage G, Berglundh T, Chapple ILC, Jepsen S, Kornman KS, Mealey BL, Papapanou PN, Sanz M, Tonetti MS. A new classification scheme for periodontal and peri-implant diseases and conditions – Introduction and key changes from the 1999 classification. J Clin Periodontol. **2018** Jun; 45 Suppl 20: S1–S8. doi: 10.1111/jcpe.12935.

Chackartchi T, Romanos GE, Sculean A. Soft tissue-related complications and management around dental implants. Periodontol 2000. **2019** Oct; 81(1): 124–138. doi: 10.1111/prd.12287.

Chambrone L, Tatakis DN. Periodontal soft tissue root coverage procedures: a systematic review from the AAP Regeneration Workshop. J Periodontol. **2015** Feb; 86 (2 Suppl): S8–S51. doi: 10.1902/jop.2015.130674.

Chan D, Pelekos G, Ho D, Cortellini P, Tonetti MS. The depth of the implant mucosal tunnel modifies the development and resolution of experimental peri-implant mucositis: A case-control study. J Clin Periodontol. **2019** Feb; 46(2): 248–255. doi: 10.1111/jcpe.13066.

Chappuis V, Buser R, Brägger U, Bornstein MM, Salvi GE, Buser D. Long-term outcomes of dental implants with a titanium plasma-sprayed surface: a 20-year prospective case series study in partially edentulous patients. Clin Implant Dent Relat Res. **2013** Dec; 15(6): 780–790. doi: 10.1111/cid.12056.

Chappuis V, Araújo MG, Buser D. Clinical relevance of dimensional bone and soft tissue alterations post-extraction in esthetic sites. Periodontol 2000. **2017** Feb;73(1): 73–83. doi: 10.1111/prd.12167. (**a**)

Chappuis V, Martin W. ITI Treatment Guide Vol. 10: Implant therapy in the esthetic zone: current treatment modalities and materials for single-tooth repacements. Buser D, Chen S, Wismeijer D (eds). Chicago: Quintessence Publishing. **2017**. (**b**)

Chappuis V, Rahman L, Buser R, Janner SFM, Belser UC, Buser D. Effectiveness of contour augmentation with guided bone regeneration: 10-year results. J Dent Res. **2018 Mar**; 97(3): 266–274. doi: 10.1177/0022034517737755.

Chen ST, Darby IB, Reynolds EC. A prospective clinical study of non-submerged immediate implants: clinical outcomes and esthetic results. Clin Oral Implants Res. **2007** Oct; 18(5): 552–462. doi: 10.1111/j.1600-0501.2007.01388.x.

Chen ST, Darby IB, Reynolds EC, Clement JG. Immediate implant placement postextraction without flap elevation. J Periodontol. 2009 Jan; 80(1): 163–172. doi: 10.1902/jop.2009.080243.

Chen ST, Buser D. Esthetic outcomes following immediate and early implant placement in the anterior maxilla--a systematic review. Int J Oral Maxillofac Implants. **2014**; 29 Suppl: 186–215. doi: 10.11607/jomi.2014suppl.g3.3.

Chung DM, Oh TJ, Shotwell JL, Misch CE, Wang HL. Significance of keratinized mucosa in maintenance of dental implants with different surfaces. J Periodontol. **2006** Aug; 77(8): 1410–1420. doi: 10.1902/jop.2006.050393.

Cochran DL, Hermann JS, Schenk RK, Higginbottom FL, Buser D. Biologic width around titanium implants. A histometric analysis of the implanto-gingival junction around unloaded and loaded nonsubmerged implants in the canine mandible. J Periodontol. **1997** Feb; 68(2): 186–198. doi: 10.1902/jop.1997.68.2.186.

Cortellini P, Pini Prato G. Coronally advanced flap and combination therapy for root coverage. Clinical strategies based on scientific evidence and clinical experience. Periodontol 2000. **2012** Jun; 59(1): 158–184. doi: 10.1111/j.1600-0757.2011.00434.x.

Cortellini P, Bissada NF. Mucogingival conditions in the natural dentition: Narrative review, case definitions, and diagnostic considerations. J Periodontol. **2018** Jun; 89 Suppl 1: S204–S213. doi: 10.1002/JPER.16-0671.

Cosgarea R, Gasparik C, Dudea D, Culic B, Dannewitz B, Sculean A. Peri-implant soft tissue colour around titanium and zirconia abutments: a prospective randomized controlled clinical study. Clin Oral Implants Res. **2015** May; 26(5): 537–544. doi: 10.1111/clr.12440.

Cosyn J, Hooghe N, De Bruyn H. A systematic review on the frequency of advanced recession following single immediate implant treatment. J Clin Periodontol. **2012** Jun; 39(6): 582–589. doi: 10.1111/j.1600-051X.2012.01888.x.

Cosyn J, De Bruyn H, Cleymaet R. Soft tissue preservation and pink aesthetics around single immediate implant restorations: a 1-year prospective study. Clin Implant Dent Relat Res. **2013** Dec; 15(6): 847–857. doi: 10.1111/j.1708-8208.2012.00448.x.

Cosyn J, De Lat L, Seyssens L, Doornewaard R, Deschepper E, Vervaeke S. The effectiveness of immediate implant placement for single tooth replacement compared to delayed implant placement: A systematic review and meta-analysis. J Clin Periodontol. **2019** Jun; 46 Suppl 21: 224–241. doi: 10.1111/jcpe.13054.

Crespi R, Capparè P, Gherlone E. A 4-year evaluation of the peri-implant parameters of immediately loaded implants in fresh extraction sockets. J Periodontol. **2010** Nov; 81(11): 1629–1634. doi: 10.1902/jop.2010.100115.

De Bruyckere T, Eeckhout C, Eghbali A, Younes F, Vandekerckhove P, Cleymaet R, Cosyn J. A randomized controlled study comparing guided bone regeneration with connective tissue graft to re-establish convexity at the buccal aspect of single implants: A one-year CBCT analysis. J Clin Periodontol. **2018** Nov; 45(11): 1375–1387. doi: 10.1111/jcpe.13006.

de Lange G. Aesthetic and prosthetic principles for single tooth implant procedures: an overview. Pract Periodontics Aesthet Dent. **1995** Jan–Feb; 7(1): 51–61.

Derks J, Schaller D, Håkansson J, Wennström JL, Tomasi C, Berglundh T. Effectiveness of implant therapy analyzed in a Swedish population: prevalence of peri-implantitis. J Dent Res. **2016** Jan; 95(1): 43–49. doi: 10.1177/0022034515608832.

Dierens M, Vandeweghe S, Kisch J, Nilner K, De Bruyn H. Long-term follow-up of turned single implants placed in periodontally healthy patients after 16–22 years: radiographic and peri-implant outcome. J Periodontol. **2013** Jul; 84(7): 880–894. doi: 10.1902/jop.2012.120187.

Dolt AH, Robbins W. Altered passive eruption: An etiology of short clinical crowns. Quintessence Int. **1997** Jun; 28(6): 363–372.

Dordick B, Coslet JG, Seibert JS. Clinical evaluation of free autogenous gingival grafts placed on alveolar bone. Part II. Coverage of nonpathologic dehiscences and fenestrations. J Periodontol. **1976**; 47(10): 568 – 573. doi:10.1902/jop.1976.47.10.568.

Edel A. Clinical evaluation of free connective tissue grafts used to increase the width of keratinised gingiva. J Clin Periodontol. **1974**; 1(4): 185 – 196. doi: 10.1111/j.1600-051x.1974.tb01257.x.

Esposito M, Grusovin MG, Kwan S, Worthington HV, Coulthard P. Interventions for replacing missing teeth: bone augmentation techniques for dental implant treatment. Cochrane Database Syst Rev. **2008** Jul; 16(3): CD003607. doi: 10.1002/14651858. CD003607.pub3.

Evans CD, Chen ST. Esthetic outcomes of immediate implant placements. Clin Oral Implants Res. **2008** Jan; 19(1): 73 – 80. doi: 10.1111/j.1600-0501.2007.01413.x.

Evian CI, Cutler SA, Rosenberg ES, Shah RK. Altered passive eruption: the undiagnosed entity. J Am Dent Assoc. **1993** Oct; 124(10): 107 – 110. doi: 10.14219/jada.archive.1993.0208.

Farina R, Filippi M, Brazzioli J, Tomasi C, Trombelli L. Bleeding on probing around dental implants: a retrospective study of associated factors. J Clin Periodontol. **2017** Jan; 44(1): 115 – 122. doi: 10.1111/jcpe.12647.

Fenner N, Hämmerle CH, Sailer I, Jung RE. Long-term clinical, technical, and esthetic outcomes of all-ceramic vs. titanium abutments on implant supporting single-tooth reconstructions after at least 5 years. Clin Oral Implants Res. **2016** Jun; 27(6): 716 – 723. doi: 10.1111/clr.12654.

Ferguson SJ, Broggini N, Wieland M, de Wild M, Rupp F, Geis-Gerstorfer J, Cochran DL, Buser D. Biomechanical evaluation of the interfacial strength of a chemically modified sandblasted and acid-etched titanium surface. J Biomed Mater Res A. **2006** Aug; 78(2) :291 – 297. doi: 10.1002/jbm.a.30678.

Ferreira Borges P, Dragoo M. Reactions of periodontal tissues to biologic implant abutments. Clinical and histologic evaluation (a pilot study). Journal GABD Online. **2010**; 5: 15 – 23.

Fickl S. Peri-implant mucosal recession: Clinical significance and therapeutic opportunities. Quintessence Int. **2015** Sep; 46(8): 671 – 676. doi: 10.3290/j. qi.a34397.

Fontana F, Maschera E, Rocchietta I, Simion M. Clinical classification of complications in guided bone regeneration procedures by means of a nonresorbable membrane. Int J Periodontics Restorative Dent. **2011** Jun; 31(3): 265 – 273.

Frisch E, Ziebolz D, Vach K, Ratka-Krüger P. The effect of keratinized mucosa width on peri-implant outcome under supportive postimplant therapy. Clin Implant Dent Relat Res. **2015** Jan; 17 Suppl 1: e236 – e244. doi: 10.1111/cid.12187.

Froum SJ, Khouly I, Tarnow DP, Froum S, Rosenberg E, Corby P, Kye W, Elian N, Schoor R, Cho SC. The use of a xenogeneic collagen matrix at the time of implant placement to increase the volume of buccal soft tissue. Int J Periodontics Restorative Dent. **2015** Mar – Apr; 35(2): 179 – 189. doi: 10.11607/prd.2226.

Fürhauser R, Florescu D, Benesch T, Haas R, Mailath G, Watzek G. Evaluation of soft tissue around single-tooth implant crowns: the pink esthetic score. Clin Oral Implants Res. **2005** Dec; 16(6): 639 – 644. doi: 10.1111/j.1600-0501.2005.01193.x.

Garber D. The esthetic dental implant: letting restoration be the guide. J Oral Implantol. **1996**; 22(1): 45 – 50.

Giannobile WV, Lang NP. Are dental implants a panacea or should we better strive to save teeth? J Dent Res. **2016** Jan; 95(1): 5 – 6. doi: 10.1177/0022034515618942.

Giannobile WV, Jung RE, Schwarz F; Groups of the 2nd Osteology Foundation Consensus Meeting. Evidence-based knowledge on the aesthetics and maintenance of peri-implant soft tissues: Osteology Foundation Consensus Report Part 1—Effects of soft tissue augmentation procedures on the maintenance of peri-implant soft tissue health. Clin Oral Implants Res. **2018** Mar; 29 Suppl 15: 7 – 10. doi: 10.1111/clr.13110.

Glauser R, Sailer I, Wohlwend A, Studer S, Schibli M, Schärer P. Experimental zirconia abutments for implant-supported single-tooth restorations in esthetically demanding regions: 4-year results of a prospective clinical study. Int J Prosthodont. **2004** May – Jun; 17(3): 285 – 290.

Glauser R, Schüpbach P, Gottlow J, Hämmerle CH. Periimplant soft tissue barrier at experimental one-piece implants with different surface topography in humans: A light-microscopic overview and histometric analysis. Clin Implant Dent Relat Res. **2005**; 7 Suppl 1: S44 – S51. doi: 10.1111/j.1708-8208.2005. tb00074.x.

Glenny AM, Esposito M, Coulthard P, Worthington HV. The assessment of systematic reviews in dentistry. Eur J Oral Sci. **2003**; 111(2): 85 – 92. doi: 10.1034/j.1600-0722.2003.00013.x.

Gobbato L, Avila-Ortiz G, Sohrabi K, Wang CW, Karimbux N. The effect of keratinized mucosa width on peri-implant health: a systematic review. Int J Oral Maxillofac Implants. **2013** Nov – Dec; 28(6): 1536 – 1545. doi: 10.11607/jomi.3244.

Godat MS, Gruen TD, Miller PD, Craddock RD. Use of tuberosity connective tissue for root coverage and ridge augmentation: backgrounds and technique. Compend Contin Educ Dent. **2018** Sep;39(8): 533 – 539.

Grischke J, Karch A, Wenzlaff A, Foitzik MM, Stiesch M, Eberhard J. Keratinized mucosa width is associated with severity of peri-implant mucositis. A cross-sectional study. Clin Oral Implants Res. **2019** May; 30(5): 457 – 465. doi: 10.1111/clr.13432.

Grossberg DE. Interimplant papilla reconstruction: assessment of soft tissue changes and results of 12 consecutive cases. J Periodontol. **2001** Jul; 72(7): 958 – 962. doi: 10.1902/jop.2001.72.7.958.

Hämmerle CH, Jung RE, Feloutzis A. A systematic review of the survival of implants in bone sites augmented with barrier membranes (guided bone regeneration) in partially edentulous patients. J Clin Periodontol. **2002**; 29 Suppl 3: 226 – 231. doi: 10.1034/j.1600-051x.29.s3.14.x

Hämmerle CH, Jung RE. Bone augmentation by means of barrier membranes. Periodontol 2000. **2003**; 33: 36 – 53.

Hämmerle CH, Chen ST, Wilson TG Jr. Consensus statements and recommended clinical procedures regarding the placement of implants in extraction sockets. Int J Oral Maxillofac Implants. **2004**; 19 Suppl: 26 – 28.

Hämmerle CHF, Tarnow D. The etiology of hard- and soft-tissue deficiencies at dental implants: A narrative review. J Clin Periodontol. **2018** Jun; 45 Suppl 20: S267 – S277. doi: 10.1111/jcpe.12955.

Hanser T, Khoury F. Alveolar ridge contouring with free connective tissue graft at implant placement: a 5-year consecutive clinical study. Int J Periodontics Restorative Dent. **2016** Jul – Aug; 36(4): 465 – 473. doi: 10.11607/prd.2730.

Happe A, Stimmelmayr M, Schlee M, Rothamel D. Surgical management of peri-implant soft tissue color mismatch caused by shine-through effects of restorative materials: one-year follow-up. Int J Periodontics Restorative Dent. **2013** Jan – Feb; 33(1): 81 – 88. doi: 10.11607/prd.1344.

Harris RJ. The connective tissue and partial thickness double pedicle graft: A predictable method of obtaining root coverage. J Periodontol. **1992** May; 63(5): 477 – 486. doi: 10.1902/jop.1992.63.5.477.

Harris RJ. Soft tissue ridge augmentation with an acellular dermal matrix. Int J Periodontics Restorative Dent. **2003** Feb; 23(1): 87 – 92.

Heitz-Mayfield LJA, Lang NP. Antimicrobial treatment of peri-implant disease. Int J Oral Maxillofac Implants. **2004**; 19 Suppl: 128 – 139.

Heitz-Mayfield LJA, Aaboe M, Araújo M, Carrión JB, Cavalcanti R, Cionca N, Cochran D, Darby I, Funakoshi E, Gierthmuehlen PC, Hashim D, Jahangiri L, Kwon Y, Lambert F, Layton DM, Lorenzana ER, McKenna G, Mombelli A, Müller F, Roccuzzo M, Salvi GE, Schimmel M, Srinivasan M, Tomasi C, Yeo A. Group 4 ITI Consensus Report: Risks and biologic complications associated with implant dentistry. Clin Oral Implants Res. **2018** Oct; 29 Suppl 16: 351 – 358. doi: 10.1111/clr.13307.

Heitz-Mayfield LJA, Salvi GE, Mombelli A, Loup PJ, Heitz F, Kruger E, Lang NP. Supportive peri-implant therapy following anti-infective surgical peri-implantitis treatment: 5-year survival and success. Clin Oral Implants Res. **2018** Jan; 29(1): 1 – 6. doi: 10.1111/ clr.12910. (**a**)

Herford AS, Akin L, Cicciu M, Maiorana C, Boyne PJ. Use of a porcine collagen matrix as an alternative to autogenous tissue for grafting oral soft tissue defects. J Oral Maxillofac Surg. **2010** Jul; 68(7): 1463 – 1470. doi: 10.1016/j.joms.2010.02.054.

Hermann JS, Buser D, Schenk RK, Higginbottom FL, Cochran DL. Biologic width around titanium implants. A physiologically formed and stable dimension over time. Clin Oral Implants Res. **2000** Feb; 11(1): 1 – 11. doi: 10.1034/j.1600-0501.2000.011001001.x.

Hermann JS, Buser D, Schenk RK, Schoolfield JD, Cochran DL. Biologic width around one- and two-piece titanium implants. Clin Oral Implants Res. **2001** Dec; 12(6): 559 – 571. doi: 10.1034/j.1600-0501.2001.120603.x.

Hidaka T, Ueno D. Mucosal dehiscence coverage for dental implant using split pouch technique: a two-stage approach [corrected]. J Periodontal Implant Sci. **2012** Jun; 42(3): 105 – 109. doi: 10.5051/jpis.2012.42.3.105.

Hinds KF. Custom impression coping for an exact registration of the healed tissue in the esthetic implant restoration. Int J Periodontics Restorative Dent. **1997** Dec; 17(6): 584 – 591.

Hofmänner P, Alessandri R, Laugisch O, Aroca S, Salvi GE, Stavropoulos A, Sculean A. Predictability of surgical techniques used for coverage of multiple adjacent gingival recessions—a systematic review. Quintessence Int. **2012** Jul – Aug: 43(7): 545 – 554

Hürzeler MB, Weng D. A single-incision technique to harvest subepithelial connective tissue grafts from the palate. Int J Periodontics Restorative Dent. **1999** Jun; 19(3): 279 – 287.

Imberman M. Gingival augmentation with an acellular dermal matrix revisited: surgical technique for gingival grafting. Pract Proced Aesthet Dent. **2007** Mar; 19(2): 123 – 128.

Ioannidis A, Cathomen E, Jung RE, Fehmer V, Hüsler J, Thoma DS. Discoloration of the mucosa caused by different restorative materials - a spectrophotometric in vitro study. Clin Oral Implants Res. **2017** Sep; 28(9): 1133 – 1138. doi: 10.1111/clr.12928.

Iorio-Siciliano V, Blasi A, Sammartino G, Salvi GE, Sculean A. Soft tissue stability related to mucosal recession at dental implants: a systematic review. Quintessence Int. **2020**; 51(1): 28 – 36. doi: 10.3290/j.qi.a43048.

Jensen SS, Terheyden H. Bone augmentation procedures in localized defects in the alveolar ridge: clinical results with different bone grafts and bone-substitute materials. Int J Oral Maxillofac Implants. **2009**;24 Suppl: 218 – 236.

Jepsen S, Berglundh T, Genco R. Aass AM, Demirel K, Derks J, Figuero E, Giovannoli JL, Goldstein M, Lambert F, Ortiz-Vigon A, Polyzois I, Salvi GE, Schwarz F, Serino G, Tomasi C, Zitzmann NU. Primary prevention of peri-implantitis: managing peri-implant mucositis. J Clin Periodontol. **2015** Apr; 42 Suppl 16: S152 – S157. doi: 10.1111/jcpe.12369.

Jepsen S, Schwarz F, Cordaro L, Derks J, Hämmerle CHF, Heitz-Mayfield LJ, Hernández-Alfaro F, Meijer HJA, Naenni N, Ortiz-Vigón A, Pjetursson B, Raghoebar GM, Renvert S, Rocchietta I, Roccuzzo M, Sanz-Sánchez I, Simion M, Tomasi C, Trombelli L, Urban I. Regeneration of alveolar ridge defects. Consensus report of group 4 of the 15th European Workshop on Periodontology on Bone Regeneration. J Clin Periodontol. **2019** Jun; 46 Suppl 21: 277 – 286. doi: 10.1111/jcpe.13121.

Jung RE, Siegenthaler DW, Hämmerle CH. Postextraction tissue management: a soft tissue punch technique. Int J Periodontics Restorative Dent. **2004** Dec; 24(6): 545 – 553.

Jung RE, Sailer I, Hämmerle CH, Attin T, Schmidlin P. In vitro color changes of soft tissues caused by restorative materials. Int J Periodontics Restorative Dent. **2007** Jun; 27(3): 251 – 257.

Jung UW, Um YJ, Choi SH. Histologic observation of soft tissue acquired from maxillary tuberosity area for root coverage. J Periodontol. **2008** May; 79(5): 934 – 940. doi: 10.1902/jop.2008.070445.

Jung RE, Holderegger C, Sailer I, Khraisat A, Suter A, Hämmerle CH. The effect of all-ceramic and porcelain-fused-to-metal restorations on marginal peri-implant soft tissue color: a randomized controlled clinical trial. Int J Periodontics Restorative Dent. **2008** Aug; 28(4): 357 – 365.

Jung UW, Um YJ, Choi SH. Histologic observation of soft tissue acquired from maxillary tuberosity area for root coverage. J Periodontol. **2008** May; 79(5): 934 – 940. doi: 10.1902/jop.2008.070445. **(b)**

Jung RE, Hälg GA, Thoma DS, Hämmerle CH. A randomized, controlled clinical trial to evaluate a new membrane for guided bone regeneration around dental implants. Clin Oral Implants Res. **2009** Feb; 20(2): 162 – 168. doi: 10.1111/j.1600-0501.2008.01634.x. doi: 10.1111/j.1600-0501.2008.01634.x.

Mathews DP. The pediculated connective tissue graft: a technique for improving unaesthetic implant restorations. Pract Proced Aesthet Dent. **2002** Nov – Dec; 14(9): 719 – 724.

Mazzotti C, Stefanini M, Felice P, Bentivogli V, Mounssif I, Zucchelli G. Soft-tissue dehiscence coverage at peri-implant sites. Periodontol 2000. **2018** Jun; 77(1): 256 – 272. doi: 10.1111/prd.12220.

McGuire MK, Scheyer ET. Xenogeneic collagen matrix with coronally advanced flap compared to connective tissue with coronally advanced flap for the treatment of dehiscence-type recession defects. J Periodontol. **2010** Aug; 81(8): 1108 – 1117. doi: 10.1902/jop.2010.090698.

Mercado F, Hamlet S, Ivanovski S. Regenerative surgical therapy for peri-implantitis using deproteinized bovine bone mineral with 10% collagen, enamel matrix derivative and doxycycline: a prospective 3-year cohort study. Clin Oral Implants Res. **2018** Jun; 29(6): 583 – 591. doi: 10.1111/clr.13256.

Merli M, Bernardelli F, Giulianelli E, Toselli I, Mariotti G, Nieri M. Peri-implant bleeding on probing: a cross-sectional multilevel analysis of associated factors. Clin Oral Implants Res. **2017** Nov; 28(11): 1401 – 1405. doi: 10.1111/clr.13001.

Mezzomo LA, Shinkai RS, Mardas N, Donos N. Alveolar ridge preservation after dental extraction and before implant placement: a literature review. Revista Odonto Ciência. **2011**: 26(1); 77 – 83.

Miller PD Jr. A classification of marginal tissue recession. Int J Periodontics Restorative Dent. **1985**; 5(2): 8 – 13.

Mitchell R. The use of collagen in oral surgery. Ann Acad Med Singapore. **1986** Jul; 15(3): 355 – 360.

Monaco C, Evangelisti E, Scotti R, Zucchelli G, Mignani G. A fully digital approach to replicate peri-implant soft tissue contours and emergence profile in the esthetic zone. Clin Oral Implants Res. **2016** Dec; 27(12): 1511 – 1514. doi: 10.1111/clr.12599.

Monje A, Blasi G. Significance of keratinized mucosa/gingiva on peri-implant and adjacent periodontal conditions in erratic maintenance compliers. J Periodontol. **2019** May; 90(5): 445 – 453. doi: 10.1002/JPER.18-0471.

Moraschini V, Luz D, Velloso G, Barboza EDP. Quality assessment of systematic reviews of the significance of keratinized mucosa on implant health. Int J Oral Maxillofac Surg. **2017** Jun; 46(6): 774 – 781. doi: 10.1016/j.ijom.2017.02.1274.

Mühlemann S, Jung R, Thoma D. Xenografts vs. autografts for soft tissue augmentation in dental implants. Forum Implantologicum. **2012**; 2: 64 – 70.

Nanci A, Bosshardt DD. Structure of periodontal tissues in health and disease. Periodontol 2000. **2006**; 40: 11 – 28. doi: 10.1111/j.1600-0757.2005.00141.x.

Nauta A, Gurtner GC, Longaker MT. Wound healing and regenerative strategies. Oral Dis. **2011** Sep; 17(6): 541 – 549. doi: 10.1111/j.1601-0825.2011.01787.x.

Oates TW, Robinson M, Gunsolley JC. Surgical Therapies for the Treatment of Gingival Recession. A Systematic Review. Ann Periodontol. **2003**; 8(1): 303 – 320. doi: 10.1902/annals.2003.8.1.303.

Oh SL, Masri RM, Williams DA, Ji C, Romberg E. Free gingival grafts for implants exhibiting lack of keratinized mucosa: a prospective controlled randomized clinical study. J Clin Periodontol. **2017** Feb; 44(2): 195 – 203. doi: 10.1111/jcpe.12660.

Orsini M, Orsini G, Benlloch D, Aranda JJ, Lázaro P, Sanz M. Esthetic and dimensional evaluation of free connective tissue grafts in prosthetically treated patients: a 1-year clinical study. J Periodontol. **2004** Mar; 75(3): 470 – 477. doi: 10.1902/jop.2004.75.3.470.

Palmer RM, Cortellini P. Periodontal tissue engineering and regeneration: Consensus Report of the Sixth European Workshop on Periodontology. J Clin Periodontol. **2008** Sep; 35(8 Suppl): 83 – 86. doi: 10.1111/j.1600-051X.2008.01262.x.

Paniz G, Mazzocco F. Surgical-prosthetic management of facial soft tissue defects on anterior single implant-supported restorations: a clinical report. Int J Esthet Dent. Int J Esthet Dent. **2015** Summer; 10(2): 270 – 284.

Papapetros D, Vassilis K, Antonis K, Danae AA. Interim tissue changes following connective tissue grafting and two-stage implant placement. A randomized clinical trial. J Clin Periodontol. **2019** Sep; 46(9): 958 – 968. doi: 10.1111/jcpe.13159.

Papi P, Pompa G. The use of a novel porcine derived acellular dermal matrix (Mucoderm) in peri-implant soft tissue augmentation: preliminary results of a prospective pilot cohort study. Biomed Res Int. **2018** Jul 9; 2018:6406051. doi: 10.1155/2018/6406051.

Park JB. Increasing the width of keratinized mucosa around endosseous implant using acellular dermal matrix allograft. Implant Dent. **2006** Sep; 15(3): 275–281. doi: 10.1097/01.id.0000227078.70869.20.

Perussolo J, Souza AB, Matarazzo F, Oliveira RP, Araújo MG. Influence of the keratinized mucosa on the stability of peri-implant tissues and brushing discomfort: A 4-year follow-up study. Clin Oral Implants Res. **2018** Dec; 29(12): 1177–1185. doi: 10.1111/clr.13381.

Pontes AE, Ribeiro FS, Iezzi G, Piattelli A, Cirelli JA, Marcantonio E Jr. Biologic width changes around loaded implants inserted in different levels in relation to crestal bone: histometric evaluation in canine mandible. Clin Oral Implants Res. **2008** May; 19(5): 483–490. doi: 10.1111/j.1600-0501.2007.01506.x.

Puisys A, Linkevicius T. The influence of mucosal tissue thickening on crestal bone stability around bone-level implants. A prospective controlled clinical trial. Clin Oral Implants Res. **2015** Feb; 26(2): 123–129. doi: 10.1111/clr.12301.

Quirynen M, Herrera D, Teughels W, Sanz M. Implant therapy: 40 years of experience. Periodontol 2000. **2014** Oct; 66(1): 7–12. doi: 10.1111/prd.12060.

Raigrodski AJ, Hillstead MB, Meng GK, Chung KH. Survival and complications of zirconia-based fixed dental prostheses: a systematic review. J Prosthet Dent. **2012** Mar; 107(3): 170–177. doi: 10.1016/S0022-3913(12)60051-1.

Ramanauskaite A, Roccuzzo A, Schwarz F. A systematic review on the influence of the horizontal distance between two adjacent implants inserted in the anterior maxilla on the inter-implant mucosa fill. Clin Oral Implants Res. **2018** Mar; 29 Suppl 15: 62–70. doi: 10.1111/clr.13103.

Rastogi S, Modi M, Sathian B. The efficacy of collagen membrane as a biodegradable wound dressing material for surgical defects of oral mucosa: a prospective study. J Oral Maxillofac Surg. **2009** Aug; 67(8): 1600–1606. doi: 10.1016/j.joms.2008.12.020.

Renvert S, Polyzois IN. Clinical approaches to treat peri-implant mucositis and peri-implantitis. Periodontol 2000. **2015** Jun; 68(1):369–404. doi: 10.1111/prd.12069.

Roccuzzo M, Bunino M, Needleman I, Sanz M. Periodontal plastic surgery for treatment of localized gingival recessions: a systematic review. Journal of Clinical Periodontology. **2002**; 29 Suppl 3: 178–194. doi: 10.1034/j.1600-051x.29.s3.11.x.

Roccuzzo M, Bonino F, Bonino L, Dalmasso P. Surgical therapy of peri-implantitis lesions by means of a bovine-derived xenograft: comparative results of a prospective study on two different implant surfaces. J Clin Periodontol. **2011** Aug; 38(8): 738–745. doi: 10.1111/j.1600-051X.2011.01742.x.

Roccuzzo M, Bonino L, Dalmasso P, Aglietta M. Long-term results of a three arms prospective cohort study on implants in periodontally compromised patients: 10-year data around sandblasted and acid-etched (SLA) surface. Clin Oral Implants Res. **2014** Oct; 25(10): 1105–1112. doi: 10.1111/clr.12227. (**a**)

Roccuzzo M, Gaudioso L, Bunino M, Dalmasso P. Surgical treatment of buccal soft tissue recessions around single implants: 1-year results from a prospective pilot study. Clin Oral Implants Res. **2014** Jun; 25(6): 641–646. doi: 10.1111/clr.12149. (**b**)

Roccuzzo M, Gaudioso L, Bunino M, Dalmasso P. Long-term stability of soft tissues following alveolar ridge preservation: 10-year results of a prospective study around nonsubmerged implants. Int J Periodontics Restorative Dent. **2014** Nov–Dec; 34(6): 795–804. doi: 10.11607/prd.2133. (c)

Roccuzzo M, Grasso G, Dalmasso P. Keratinized mucosa around implants in partially edentulous posterior mandible: 10-year results of a prospective comparative study. Clin Oral Implants Res. **2016** Apr; 27(4): 491–496. doi: 10.1111/clr.12563.

Roccuzzo M, Savoini M, Dalmasso P, Ramieri G. Long-term outcomes of implants placed after vertical alveolar ridge augmentation in partially edentulous patients: a 10-year prospective clinical study. Clin Oral Implants Res. **2017** Oct; 28(10): 1204–1210. doi: 10.1111/clr.12941.

Roccuzzo M, Pittoni D, Roccuzzo A, Charrier L, Dalmasso P. Surgical treatment of peri-implantitis intrabony lesions by means of deproteinized bovine bone mineral with 10% collagen: 7-year-results. Clin Oral Implants Res. **2017** Dec;28(12):1577-1583. doi: 10.1111/clr.13028.

Roccuzzo M, Dalmasso P, Pittoni D, Roccuzzo A. Treatment of buccal soft tissue dehiscence around single implant: 5-year results from a prospective study. Clin Oral Investig. **2019** Apr; 23(4): 1977 – 1983. doi: 10.1007/s00784-018-2634-4.

Rojo E, Stroppa G, Sanz-Martín I, Gonzalez-Martín O, Alemany AS, Nart J. Soft tissue volume gain around dental implants using autogenous subepithelial connective tissue grafts harvested from the lateral palate or tuberosity area. A randomized controlled clinical study. J Clin Periodontol. **2018** Apr; 45(4): 495 – 503. doi: 10.1111/jcpe.12869.

Romanos G, Grizas E, Nentwig GH. Association of keratinized mucosa and periimplant soft tissue stability around implants with platform switching. Implant Dent. **2015** Aug; 24(4): 422 – 426. doi: 10.1097/ID.0000000000000274.

Rompen E, Domken O, Degidi M, Pontes AE, Piattelli A. The effect of material characteristics, of surface topography and of implant components and connections on soft tissue integration: a literature review. Clin Oral Implants Res. **2006** Oct; 17 Suppl 2: 55 – 67. doi: 10.1111/j.1600-0501.2006.01367.x.

Rossi S, Tirri T, Paldan H, Kuntsi-Vaattovaara H, Tulamo R, Närhi T. Peri-implant tissue response to TiO2 surface modified implants. Clin Oral Implants Res. **2008** Apr; 19(4): 348 – 355. doi: 10.1111/j.1600-0501.2007.01478.x.

Saffar JL, Lasfargues JJ, Cherruau M. Alveolar bone and the alveolar process: the socket that is never stable. Periodontol 2000. **1997** Feb; 13: 76 – 90. doi: 10.1111/j.1600-0757.1997.tb00096.x.

Sailer I, Makarov NA, Thoma DS, Zwahlen M, Pjetursson BE. All-ceramic or metal-ceramic tooth-supported fixed dental prostheses (FDPs)? A systematic review of the survival and complication rates. Part I: Single crowns (SCs). Dent Mater. **2015** Jun; 31/6), 603 – 623. doi: 10.1016/j.dental.2015.02.011.

Salvi GE, Aglietta M, Eick S, Sculean A, Lang NP, Ramseier CA. Reversibility of experimental peri-implant mucositis compared with experimental gingivitis in humans. Clin Oral Implants Res. **2012** Feb; 23(2): 182 – 190. doi: 10.1111/j.1600-0501.2011.02220.x.

Sanz M, Lorenzo R, Aranda JJ, Martin C, Orsini M. Clinical evaluation of a new collagen matrix (Mucograft prototype) to enhance the width of keratinized tissue in patients with fixed prosthetic restorations: a randomized prospective clinical trial. J Clin Periodontol. **2009** Oct; 36(10): 868 – 876. doi: 10.1111/j.1600-051X.2009.01460.x.

Sanz M, Dahlin C, Apatzidou D, Artzi Z, Bozic D, Calciolari E, De Bruyn H, Dommisch H, Donos N, Eickholz P, Ellingsen JE, Haugen HJ, Herrera D, Lambert F, Layrolle P, Montero E, Mustafa K, Omar O, Schliephake H. Biomaterials and regenerative technologies used in bone regeneration in the craniomaxillofacial region: Consensus report of group 2 of the 15th European Workshop on Periodontology on Bone Regeneration. J Clin Periodontol. **2019** Jun; 46 Suppl 21: 82 – 91. doi: 10.1111/jcpe.13123.

Sanz-Martín I, Rojo E, Maldonado E, Stroppa G, Nart J, Sanz M. Structural and histological differences between connective tissue grafts harvested from the lateral palatal mucosa or from the tuberosity area. Clin Oral Investig. **2019** Feb; 23(2): 957 – 964. doi: 10.1007/s00784-018-2516-9.

Schallhorn RA, McClain PK, Charles A, Clem D, Newman MG. Evaluation of a porcine collagen matrix used to augment keratinized tissue and increase soft tissue thickness around existing dental implants. Int J Periodontics Restorative Dent. **2015** Jan – Feb; 35(1): 99 – 103. doi: 10.11607/prd.1888.

Schluger S, Yuodelis R, Page R. Resective periodontal surgery in pocket elimination. In: Periodontal disease. Basic phenomena, clinical management, and occlusal and restorative interrelationships (chapter 22). Philadelphia: Lea & Febiger. **1977;** 470 – 519.

Schmitt CM, Moest T, Lutz R, Wehrhan F, Neukam FW, Schlegel KA. Long-term outcomes after vestibuloplasty with a porcine collagen matrix (Mucograft®) versus the free gingival graft: a comparative prospective clinical trial. Clin Oral Implants Res. **2016** Nov; 27(11): e125 – e133. doi: 10.1111/clr.12575.

Schou S, Holmstrup P, Hjorting-Hansen E, et al. Plaque-induced marginal tissue reactions of osseointegrated oral implants: a review of the literature. Clin Oral Implants Res. **1992** Dec; 3(4): 149–161. doi: 10.1034/j.1600-0501.1992.030401.x.

Schroeder HE, Listgarten MA. The gingival tissues: the architecture of periodontal protection. Periodontol 2000. **1997** Feb; 13: 91–120. doi: 10.1111/j.1600-0757.1997.tb00097.x.

Schrott AR, Jimenez M, Hwang JW, Fiorellini J, Weber HP. Five year evaluation on the influence of keratinized mucosa on peri-implant soft health and stability around implants supporting full-arch mandibular fixed prostheses. Clin Oral Implants Res. **2009** Oct; 20(10): 1170–1177. doi: 10.1111/j.1600-0501.2009.01795.x.

Schwarz F, Ferrari D, Herten M, Mihatovic I, Wieland M, Sager M, Becker J. Effects of surface hydrophilicity and microtopography on early stages of soft and hard tissue integration at non-submerged titanium implants: an immunohistochemical study in dogs. J Periodontol. **2007** Nov; 78(11): 2171–2184. doi: 10.1902/jop.2007.070157.

Schwarz F, Sahm N, Iglhaut G, Becker J. Impact of the method of surface debridement and decontamination on the clinical outcome following combined surgical therapy of peri-implantitis: a randomized controlled clinical study. J Clin Periodontol. **2011** Mar; 38(3): 276–284. doi: 10.1111/j.1600-051X.2010.01690.x.

Schwarz F, John G, Mainusch S, Sahm N, Becker J. Combined surgical therapy of peri-implantitis evaluating two methods of surface debridement and decontamination. A two-year follow-up report. J Clin Periodontol. **2012** Aug; 39(8): 789–797. doi: 10.1111/j.1600-051X.2012.01867.x.

Schwarz F, Derks J, Monje A, Wang H-L. Peri-implantitis. J Periodontol. **2018** Jun; 89 Suppl 1: S267–S290. doi: 10.1002/JPER.16-0350.

Sculean A, Gruber R, Bosshardt DD. Soft tissue wound healing at teeth and dental implants. J Clin Periodontol. **2014** Apr; 41 Suppl 15: S6–S22. doi: 10.1111/jcpe.12206.(a)

Sculean A, Cosgarea R, Stähli A, Katsaros C, Arweiler NB, Brecx M, Deppe H. The modified coronally advanced tunnel combined with an enamel matrix derivative and subepithelial connective tissue graft for the treatment of isolated mandibular Miller Class I and II gingival recessions: a report of 16 cases. Quintessence Int. **2014** Nov–Dec; 45(10): 829–835. doi: 10.3290/j.qi.a32636.(b)

Sculean A, Cosgarea R, Stähli A, Katsaros C, Arweiler NB, Miron RJ, Deppe H. Treatment of multiple adjacent maxillary Miller Class I, II, and III gingival recessions with the modified coronally advanced tunnel, enamel matrix derivative, and subepithelial connective tissue graft: A report of 12 cases. Quintessence Int. **2016**; 47(8): 653–659. doi: 10.3290/j.qi.a36562.

Sculean A, Chappuis V, Cosgarea R. Coverage of mucosal recessions at dental implants. Periodontol 2000. **2017** Feb; 73(1): 134–140. doi: 10.1111/prd.12178.(a)

Sculean A, Cosgarea R, Katsaros C, Arweiler NB, Miron RJ, Deppe H. Treatment of single and multiple Miller Class I and III gingival recessions at crown-restored teeth in maxillary esthetic areas. Quintessence Int. 2017; 48(10): 777–782. doi: 10.3290/j.qi.a39031. (b)

Sculean A, Allen EP. The laterally closed tunnel for the treatment of deep isolated mandibular recessions: surgical technique and a report of 24 cases. Int J Periodontics Restorative Dent. **2018** Jul–Aug; 38(4): 479–487. doi: 10.11607/prd.3680.

Sculean A, Romanos G, Schwarz F, Ramanauskaite A, Keeve PL, Khoury F, Koo KT, Cosgarea R. Soft-tissue management a spart oft he surgical treatment of periimplantitis: a narrative review. Implant Dent. **2019** Apr; 28(2): 210–216. doi: 10.1097/ID.0000000000000870.

Seibert J, Salama H. Alveolar ridge preservation and reconstruction. Periodontol 2000. **1996** Jun; 11: 69–84. doi: 10.1111/j.1600-0757.1996.tb00185.x.

Shahidi P, Jacobson Z, Dibart S, Pourati J, Nunn ME, Barouch K, Van Dyke TE. Efficacy of a new papilla generation technique in implant dentistry: a preliminary study. Int J Oral Maxillofac Implants. **2008** Sep–Oct; 23(5): 926–934.

Shea BJ, Grimshaw JM, Wells GA, Boers M, Andersson N, Hamel C, Porter AC, Tugwell P, Moher D, Bouter LM. Development of AMSTAR: a measurement tool to assess the methodological quality of systematic reviews. BMC Med Res Methodol. **2007** Feb 15; 7: 10. doi: 10.1186/1471-2288-7-10.

Shibli JA, d'Avila S, Marcantonio E Jr. Connective tissue graft to correct peri-implant soft tissue margin: A clinical report. J Prosthet Dent. **2004** Feb; 91(2): 119–122. doi: 10.1016/j.prosdent.2003.09.017.

Shibli JA, d'Avila S. Restoration of the soft-tissue margin in single-tooth implant in the anterior maxilla. J Oral Implantol. **2006**; 32(6): 286–290. doi: 10.1563/0-790.1.

Sicilia A, Botticelli D. Computer-guided implant therapy and soft- and hard-tissue aspects. The Third EAO Consensus Conference 2012. Clin Oral Implants Res. **2012** Oct; 23 Suppl 6: 157–161. doi: 10.1111/j.1600-0501.2012.02553.x.

Silverstein L, Lefkove M. The use of the subepithelial connective tissue graft to enhance both the aesthetics and periodontal contours surrounding dental implants. J Oral Implantol. **1994**; 20(2): 135–138.

Simion M, Fontana F, Rasperini G, Maiorana C. Vertical ridge augmentation by expanded-polytetrafluoroethylene membrane and a combination of intraoral autogenous bone graft and deproteinized anorganic bovine bone (Bio-Oss). Clin Oral Implants Res. **2007** Oct; 18(5): 620–629. doi: 10.1111/j.1600-0501.2007.01389.x.

Simons AM, Darany DG, Giordano JR. The use of free gingival grafts in the treatment of peri-implant soft tissue complications: clinical report. Implant Dent. **1993** Spring; 2(1): 27–30. doi: 10.1097/00008505-199304000-00006.

Souza AB, Tormena M, Matarazzo F, Araújo MG. The influence of peri-implant keratinized mucosa on brushing discomfort and peri-implant tissue health. Clin Oral Implants Res. **2016** Jun; 27(6): 650–655. doi: 10.1111/clr.12703.

Speroni S, Cicciù M, Maridati P, Grossi GB, Maiorana C. Clinical investigation of mucosal thickness stability after soft tissue grafting around implants: a 3-year retrospective study. Indian J Dent Res. **2010** Oct–Dec; 21(4): 474–479. doi: 10.4103/0970-9290.74208.

Spray JR, Black CG, Morris HF, Ochi S. The influence of bone thickness on facial marginal bone response: stage 1 placement through stage 2 uncovering. Ann Periodontol. **2000** Dec; 5(1): 119–128. doi: 10.1902/annals.2000.5.1.119.

Stefanini M, Felice P, Mazzotti C, Marzadori M, Gherlone EF, Zucchelli G. Transmucosal implant placement with submarginal connective tissue graft in area of shallow buccal bone dehiscence: a three-year follow-up case series. Int J Periodontics Restorative Dent. **2016** Sep–Oct; 36(5): 621–630. doi: 10.11607/prd.2537.

Strub JR, Gaberthuel TW, Grunder U. The role of attached gingiva in the health of peri-implant tissue in dogs. 1. Clinical findings. Int J Periodontics Restorative Dent. **1991**; 11(4): 317–333.

Studer SP, Allen EP, Rees TC, Kouba A. The thickness of masticatory mucosa in the human hard palate and tuberosity as potential donor sites for ridge augmentation procedures. J Periodontol. **1997** Feb; 68(2): 145–151. doi: 10.1902/jop.1997.68.2.145.

Suárez-López Del Amo F, Lin GH, Monje A, Galindo-Moreno P, Wang HL. Influence of soft tissue thickness on peri-implant marginal bone loss. A systematic review and meta-analysis. J Periodontol. **2016** Jun; 87(6): 690–699. doi: 10.1902/jop.2016.150571.

Subramani K, Wismeijer D. Decontamination of titanium implant surface and re-osseointegration to treat peri-implantitis: a literature review. Int J Oral Maxillofac Implants. **2012** Sep–Oct; 27(5): 1043–1054.

Sullivan HC, Atkins JH. The role of free gingival grafts in periodontal therapy. Dent Clin North Am. **1969** Jan; 13(1): 133–148.

Tarnow DP, Cho SC, Wallace SS. The effect of inter-implant distance on the height of inter-implant bone crest. J Periodontol. **2000** Apr; 71(4): 546–549. doi: 10.1902/jop.2000.71.4.546.

Tatarakis N, Gkranias N, Darbar U, Donos N. Blood flow changes using a 3D xenogeneic collagen matrix or a subepithelial connective tissue graft for root coverage procedures: a pilot study. Clin Oral Investig. **2018** May; 22(4): 1697–1705. doi: 10.1007/s00784-017-2261-5.

Tavelli L, Barootchi S, Greenwell H, Wang HL. Is a soft tissue graft harvested from the maxillary tuberosity the approach of choice in an isolated site? J Periodontol. **2019** Sug; 90(8): 821–825. doi:10.1002/JPER.18-0615.

Thoma DS, Benic GI, Zwahlen M, Hämmerle CH, Jung RE. A systematic review assessing soft tissue augmentation techniques. Clin Oral Implants Res. **2009** Sep; 20 Suppl 4: 146 – 165. doi: 10.1111/j.1600-0501.2009.01784.x.

Thoma DS, Buranawat B, Hämmerle CH, Held U, Jung RE. Efficacy of soft tissue augmentation around dental implants and in partially edentulous areas: A systematic review. J Clin Periodontol. **2014** Apr; 41 Suppl 15: S77 – S91. doi: 10.1111/jcpe.12220.

Thoma DS, Brandenberg F, Fehmer V, Knechtle N, Hämmerle CH, Sailer I. The esthetic effect of veneered zirconia abutments for single-tooth implant reconstructions: a randomized controlled clinical trial. Clin Implant Dent Relat Res. **2016** Dec; 18(6): 1210 – 1217. doi: 10.1111/cid.12388.

Thoma DS, Naenni N, Figuero E, Hämmerle CHF, Schwarz F, Jung RE, Sanz-Sánchez I. Effects of soft tissue augmentation procedures on peri-implant health or disease: A systematic review and meta-analysis. Clin Oral Implants Res. **2018** Mar; 29 Suppl 15: 32 – 49. doi: 10.1111/clr.13114.

Thoma DS, Alshihri A, Fontolliet A, Hämmerle CHF, Jung RE, Benic GI. Clinical and histologic evaluation of different approaches to gain keratinized tissue prior to implant placement in fully edentulous patients. Clin Oral Investig. **2018** Jun; 22(5): 2111 – 2119. doi: 10.1007/s00784-017-2319-4.

Thoma DS, Lim HC, Paeng KW, Kim MJ, Jung RE, Hämmerle CHF, Jung UW. Augmentation of keratinized tissue at tooth and implant sites by using autogenous grafts and collagen-based soft-tissue substitutes. J Clin Periodontol. **2020** Jan; 47(1): 64 – 71. doi: 10.1111/jcpe.13194.

Tinti C, Parma-Benfenati S. Vertical ridge augmentation: surgical protocol and retrospective evaluation of 48 consecutively inserted implants. Int J Periodontics Restorative Dent. **1998** Oct; 18(5): 434 – 443.

Tinti C, Parma-Benfenati S. Minimally invasive technique for gingival augmentation around dental implants. Int J Periodontics Restorative Dent. **2012** Apr; 32(2): 187 – 193.

Tomasi C, Tessarolo F, Caola I, Wennström J, Nollo G, Berglundh T. Morphogenesis of peri-implant mucosa revisited: an experimental study in humans. Clin Oral Implants Res. **2014** Sep; 25(9): 997 – 1003. doi: 10.1111/clr.12223.

Tonetti MS, Jung RE, Avila-Ortiz G, Blanco J, Cosyn J, Fickl S, Figuero E, Goldstein M, Graziani F, Madianos P, Molina A, Nart J, Salvi GE, Sanz-Martín I, Thoma D, Van Assche N, Vignoletti F. Management of the extraction socket and timing of implant placement: Consensus report and clinical recommendations of group 3 of the XV European Workshop in Periodontology. J Clin Periodontol. **2019** Jun; 46 Suppl 21: 183 – 194. doi: 10.1111/jcpe.13131.

Ueno D, Nagano T, Watanabe T, Shirakawa S, Yashima A, Gomi K. Effect of the keratinized mucosa width on the health status of periimplant and contralateral periodontal tissues: a cross-sectional study. Implant Dent. **2016** Dec; 25(6): 796 – 801. doi: 10.1097/ID.0000000000000483.

Venezia P, Torsello F, Cavalcanti R, D'Amato S. Retrospective analysis of 26 complete-arch implant-supported monolithic zirconia prostheses with feldspathic porcelain veneering limited to the facial surface. J Prosthet Dent. **2015** Oct; 114(4): 506 – 512. doi: 10.1016/j.prosdent.2015.02.010.

Venezia P, Torsello F, Cavalcanti R, Casiello E, Chiapasco M. Digital registration of peri-implant transmucosal portion and pontic area in the esthetic zone. J Osseointegr **2017**; 9 (4): 312 – 316. doi: 10.23805 / JO.2017.09.04.01.

Vignoletti F, Nunez J, Sanz M. Soft tissue wound healing at teeth, dental implants and the edentulous ridge when using barrier membranes, growth and differentiation factors and soft tissue substitutes. J Clin Periodontol. **2014** Apr; 41 Suppl 15: S23 – S35. doi: 10.1111/jcpe.12191.

von Arx T, Buser D. Horizontal ridge augmentation using autogenous block grafts and the guided bone regeneration technique with collagen membranes: a clinical study with 42 patients. Clin Oral Implants Res. **2006** Aug; 17(4): 359 – 366. doi: 10.1111/j.1600-0501.2005.01234.x.

Wallace SS, Froum SJ. Effect of maxillary sinus augmentation on the survival of endosseous dental implants. A systematic review. Ann Periodontol. **2003** Dec; 8(1): 328 – 343. doi: 10.1902/annals.2003.8.1.328.

Warrer K, Buser D, Lang NP, Karring T. Plaque-induced peri-implantitis in the presence or absence of keratinized mucosa. An experimental study in monkeys. Clin Oral Implants Res. **1995** Sep; 6(3): 131 – 138.

ITI International Team for Implantology